ESWARAN TAMILSELVI
VS SELVAMANI

NEXT-GENERATION DRUG DELIVERY

ESWARAN TAMILSELVI
VS SELVAMANI

NEXT-GENERATION DRUG DELIVERY

FROM EMULSIFICATION METHODS TO CLINICAL TRANSLATION

LAP LAMBERT Academic Publishing

Imprint

Cover image: www.ingimage.com

Publisher:
LAP LAMBERT Academic Publishing
is a trademark of
Dodo Books Indian Ocean Ltd. and OmniScriptum S.R.L publishing group

120 High Road, East Finchley, London, N2 9ED, United Kingdom
Str. Armeneasca 28/1, office 1, Chisinau MD-2012, Republic of Moldova, Europe
Managing Directors: Ieva Konstantinova, Victoria Ursu
info@omniscriptum.com

Printed at: see last page
ISBN: 978-620-8-44208-8

NEXT-GENERATION DRUG DELIVERY: FROM EMULSIFICATION METHODS TO CLINICAL TRANSLATION

Microsphere drug delivery system

Enhanced Stability and Sustained Activity of Drug via Emulsification-Solvent Evaporation: A Preclinical Outlook Toward Disposition Kinetics and Dosage Optimization

Tamil Selvi Eswaran*, selvamani

Department of Pharmaceutics, Karpagam College of Pharmacy, Othakalmandapam, Coimbatore-32, Tamil Nadu, India.

***Corresponding author:**

Mrs. E.Tamil Selvi, M.Pharm., Ph.D

Associate professor,

Department of Pharmaceutics,

Karpagam College of Pharmacy,

Othakalmandapam,

Coimbatore, Tamil Nadu, India.

E-mail - selvimadhu05@gmail.com

Tel: 8675165765

1. INTRODUCTION

1.1 POTENTIAL OF NOVEL DRUG DELIVERY FOR HERBAL DRUGS:

Novel drug delivery system is a novel approach to drug delivery that addresses the limitations of the traditional drug delivery systems. Our country has a vast knowledge base of Ayurveda whose potential is only being realized in the recent years. However, the drug delivery system used for administering the herbal medicine to the patient is traditional and out-of-date, resulting in reduced efficacy of the drug. If the novel drug delivery technology is applied in herbal medicine, it may help in increasing the efficacy and reducing the side effects of various herbal compounds and herbs. This is the basic idea behind incorporating novel drug delivery system and Indian Ayurvedic medicines to combat more serious diseases.

For a long time, herbal medicines were not considered for development as novel formulations owing to lack of scientific justification and processing difficulties, such as standardization, extraction and identification of individual drug components in complex polyherbal systems. However, modern phytopharmaceutical research can solve the scientific needs of herbal medicines to be incorporated in novel drug delivery system, such as nanoparticles, solid lipid nanoparticles, microspheres, magnetic microspheres, microemulsions, solid dispersions, liposomes, niosomes, proniosomes, Transdermal patches, matrix systems, etc.

The future of medicine is rooted in the past itself. In the past, almost all the medicines were from the plants; the plant being man's only chemist for ages. Herbs are staging a comeback, herbal 'renaissance' is happening all over the globe and more and more people are taking note of herbal therapies to treat various kinds of ailments in place of mainstream medicine. There are three main reasons for the popularity of herbal medicines:

- There is a growing concern over the reliance and safety if drugs and surgery.
- Modern medicine is failing to effectively treat many of the most common health conditions.
- Many natural measures are being shown to produce better results than drugs or surgery without the side effects.

1.2 HISTORY OF TRADITIONAL AND HERBAL MEDICINE:

Although written records about medicinal plants dated back at least 5,000 years to the Sumerians, who described well-established medicinal uses for such plants as laurel, caraway, and thyme, archeological studies have shown that the practice of herbal medicine dates as far back as 60,000 years ago in Iraq and 8,000 years ago in China. With the advent of western medicine (or "conventional" medicine) over the past century, herbal medicine has been challenged by practitioners of mainstream medicine because of the lack of scientific evidence in the context of contemporary medicine, despite its long history of effective use. Interestingly, things change with time.

Topical remedies anointed, bandaged, rubbed or applied to the skin are likely to have been used since the origin of man, with the practices becoming evident with the appearance of written records, such as on the clay tablets used by the Sumerians (Kramer, 1963).

A millennium and a half later, Galen (AD 129-199), a Greek physician, introduced the compounding of herbal drugs and other excipients into dosage forms. He is widely considered to be the "Father of Pharmacy" and his practices are known as 'Galenic pharmacy'.

The well-known Papyrus Eber (1550 BC), describing more than 800 prescriptions and about 700 drugs, appear to be the best pharmaceutical record from ancient times (La Wall, 1927). It contains many recipes for treating skin conditions, including burns, wounds, blisters and exudation. Other remedies are to preserve the hair, to make the hair grow, to improve the skin and to beautify the body.

1.2.1 TRADITIONAL SYSTEM OF MEDICINES:

- Ayurveda
- Unani
- Siddha
- Homeopathy

Ayurveda:

Our country has a vast knowledge base of Ayurveda whose potential is only being realized in the recent years. Ayurvedic medicine is a system of traditional medicine native to the Indian subcontinent and practiced in other parts of the world as a form of traditional medicine in Sanskrit the word Ayurveda consist of the sayus means "longevity" and veda means "related to knowledge" or "science" evolving throughout at its history ayurveda remains an influential system of medicine in South Asia the earliest literature on Indian medical practice appeared during the vedic period in India the Susruta Samhta where influential works on traditional medicine during this era Ayurveda is considered to be a form of Complementary and Alternative Medicine (CAM) in the western world where several of its methods such as the use of herbs massage and yoga are applied on their own as a form of CAM treatment.

Ayurveda is the ancient (before 2500BC) Indian system of health care involving a holistic view of man his health and illness. Ayurvedic treatment of a disease consists of salubrious use of drugs, diets, and certain practices medicinal preparation is invariably complex mixtures based mostly on plant products around 1250 plants are used various Ayurvedic preparations.

Many Indian medicinal plants have come under scientific scrutiny since the middle of the nineteenth century although in a sporadic fashion. The first significant contribution from ayurvedic material medica came with the isolation of the hypertensive alkaloids from the sarpagandha plant valued in Ayurveda for the treatment of hypertension, insomnia and insanity. This was the first important ancient modern concordance in Ayurvedic plants.

Siddha:

Siddha system is one of the oldest systems of medicine in India the term siddha means achievements and siddhars were saintly persons who achieved results in medicine eighteen siddhars were said to have contributed towards the development of this medical system. Siddha literature is in Tamil and it is practiced largely in Tamil speaking part of India and abroad the siddha system is largely therapeutic in nature.

The principles and doctorines of this system both fundamental and applied have a close similarity to Ayurveda with specialization in nitro chemistry according to this system the human body is the replica of the universe and so are the food and drugs irrespective of their origin.

Unani:

"Unani" or "Yunani medicine" is the term for Perso-Arabic traditional medicine as practiced in Mughal India and in Muslim culture in South Asia and modern Central Asia. The term Yunani means "Greek", as the Perso-Arabic system of medicine was based on the teachings of the Greek physicians Hippocrates and Galen. The Hellenistic origin of Unani medicine is still visible in its being based on the classical four humors: phlegm (balgham), blood (dam), yellow bile (safra) and black bile (sauda), but it has also been influenced by Indian and Chinese traditional systems.

Arab and Persian elaborations upon the Greek system of medicine by figures like Ibn Sina and Al-Razi influenced the early development of Unani. The medical tradition of medieval Islam was introduced to India by the 13th century with the establishment of the Delhi Sultanate and it took its own course of development during the Mughal Empire, influenced by Indian medical teachings of Sushruta and Charaka. Alauddin Khalji has several eminent physicians (Hakims) at his royal courts. This royal patronage led to the development of Unani in India, and also the creation of Unani literature.

Homeopathy:

Homeopathy is a pseudoscientific system founded by a German physician Samuel Hahnemann in 1796 is based on the idea "Like cures like" that is the substance that cause certain symptoms in healthy person can also cure those symptoms in someone who is sick. This is so called Law of Similars gives homeopathy its name "homeo" for similar "pathy" designating disease in this experiment Hahnemann developed a method of "potentizing" homeopathic remedies by diluting them in a water alcohol solution and then vigorously shaking the mixtures.

The result convinced him that a high degree of dilution not only minimizes the side effects of the remedies but also simultaneously enhances their medical efficacy homeopathic remedies have undergone proving or medical observation in which healthy individuals are given doses of undiluted homeopathic substances. Mental, emotional, and other details of the patients are most important this leads the physician to a better understanding of which remedy will best suits a particular symptom over the past 200 years, providing for almost 2000 substances have been conducted.

1.3 MICROSPHERES BASED ON HERBAL DRUGS:

Microspheres are an important part of NDDSs and have the potential to deliver drug in a controlled manner. Advancement in herbal field using novel technology for drug delivery or carriers is significantly enhanced due to its biodegradability and its nontoxic nature with minimum side effects and better therapeutic value. Encapsulated herbal compounds or herbal extracts within microspheres can be used in targeting the site of action with minimum toxicity, thus enhancing bioavailability. NDDS has helped in overcoming the issues of stability and limited absorption attributed to most of the herbal drugs, thereby opening new avenues towards the development of herbal drug delivery systems. Nowadays, with the help of the biomedical system, the use of modern medicine is associated with various side effects, and increased cost of Synthetic drugs are the factor that helps in gaining the interest on the use of traditional medicine. WHO declared that the incorrect use of herbal medicine may cause hazardous or dangerous effects and that further research is needed to ascertain its efficacy and safety. However, for delivery of herbal drugs, modifications to achieve sustained release are required so as to achieve patient compliance. Herbal medicines possess pharmacological activity due to its specific constituents or blend of constituents. The challenges encountered in the use of herbal products prevent the usage over the synthetic drugs, and achieve improved development by the use of different carrier systems such as microparticulate system, nanotechnology, liposome, and phytosomes so as to target the specific site with desired concentrations and achieve therapeutic value. Microspheres can be formulated by various natural drugs such as garlic, camptothecin, apple, tea, berries, cauliflower, onion, nuts, cabbage, turmeric, soya beans, peapods, red grapes, eucalyptus, spruce, blue berries, mulberries, peanuts.

1.4 REASON FOR THE SELECTION OF MUSA PARADISIACA LEAVES:

Banana leaves are 100% environmentally – friendly and sustainable. They will degrade just like any other plant product once they have been discarded, and they are a by – product that is continuously produced. They are cheap. It is believed that eating in banana leaf will helps in easy digestion. And it is easily available. It is said to prevent many lifestyle diseases.

1.5 MICROSPHERES:

Microspheres can be described as small particles (in 1-1000 micrometer size range) for use as carriers of drugs and other therapeutic agents consisting of proteins or synthetic polymers which are biodegradable in nature. The term microsphere describes a monolithic spherical structure with the drug or therapeutic agent distributed throughout the matrix either as a molecular dispersion or as a dispersion of particles. The behavior of the drugs in vivo can be manipulated by combining the drug to a carrier particle. The clearance kinetics, tissue distribution, metabolism i.e. kinetics and drug carrier phenomenon require a detailed understanding of the carrier interaction with cellular interaction of the drug are strongly influenced by the behavior of the carrier. The exploitation of these changes in pharmacodynamics behavior may lead to enhanced therapeutic efficiency. However, an intelligent approach to therapeutics employing and organ systems and of the limitations of the systems with respect to the formulation procedures and stability issues. There are two types

•Microcapsule

•Micrometrics.

Microcapsules are those in which entrapped substance is distinctly surrounded by distinct capsule wall and micrometrics in which entrapped substance is dispersing throughout the microsphere matrix. Solid biodegradable microspheres incorporating a drug dispersed or dissolved through particle matrix have the potential for the controlled release of drug. They are made up of polymeric, waxy, or other protective materials, that is biodegradable synthetic polymers and modified natural products.

1.5.1 Materials used in the preparation of microspheres:

The microspheres used usually are polymers. They are classified into 2 types:

A] Natural polymers

B] Synthetic polymers

1.5.1.1A] Natural Polymers:

The natural polymers that are obtained from the different sources like carbohydrates, chemically modified carbohydrate s &proteins.

- Carbohydrates: Eg: Starch, Agarose, Chitosan, Carrageenan.
- Chemically modified carbohydrates: Eg: Poly search, Poly dextran.
- Proteins: Eg: Collagen, Albumin & Gelatin.

1.5.1.2 B] Synthetic polymers:

Into 2 types the synthetic polymers are divided as

- Biodegradable polymers:

For e.g. Poly anhydrides, Lactides, Poly alkyl cyanoacrylates, Glycoside & their copolymers,

- Non-biodegradable polymers:

For e.g. PMMA [Polymethylmethacrylate], Epoxy polymers, Acrolein, Glycidyl methacrylate

1.5.2CHARACTERSTICS:

1. Microsphere size may be critical to the proper function of an assay, or it may be secondary to other characteristics. The test or assay format commonly dictate particle size, such as the use of very small spheres (~0.1- 0.4µm) to ensure satisfactory wicking in lateral flow tests, or the use of larger, cell-sized spheres (~4-10µm) for bead- based flow cytometric assays.

2. Common microsphere compositions include polystyrene (PS), poly (methyl methacrylate) (PMMA), and silica. These materials possess different physical and optical properties, which may present advantages or limitations for different applications. Polymer beads are generally hydrophobic, and as such, have high protein binding abilities. However, they often require the use of some surfactant (e.g. 0.01-0.1% Tween® 20 or SDS) in the storage buffer to ensure ease of handling. During synthesis, functional monomers may be co-polymerized with styrene or methyl methacrylate to develop beads with surface reactive groups. Functional groups may be used in covalent binding reactions, and also aid in stabilizing the suspension. Silica microspheres are inherently hydrophilic and negatively charged. Consequently, aqueous silica suspensions rarely require use of surfactants or other stabilizers. Carboxyl- and amine functionalized silica spheres are available for use in common covalent coating protocols, and

plain silica microspheres may be modified using a variety of silanes to generate functional groups or alter surface properties.

3. Many applications in the life sciences demand added properties, such as fluorescence or a visible color, or iron oxide inclusions for magnetic separations. Polymer spheres (and polymer based magnetic spheres) are often internally dyed via organic solvent swelling, and many standard products are available. Dye concentrations can be adjusted to produce beads with different intensities to meet special needs, such as Quantum Plex™ for multiplexed flow cytometric assays, or our Dragon Green or Flash Red Intensity Standards, which support imaging applications and associated instrument QC. Many surface- or internally labeled fluorescent beads are also available as specialized flow cytometry standards.

1.5.3 Advantages of microspheres over conventional dosage forms:

- Microspheres provide prolonged and constant therapeutic effect. Particle size reduction for enhancing solubility of the poorly soluble drug.
- Microspheres reduce the dosing frequency and therefore improve the patient compliance.
- Protect the drug from enzymatic and photolytic cleavage hence found to be best for drug delivery of protein.
- Microspheres provide controlled, sustained and targeted delivery of the drug. Biodegradable microspheres have the advantage over large polymer implants in that they do not require surgical procedures for implantation and removal.
- Microspheres produce more reproducible drug absorption. Drug discharge in stomach is hindered and that's why local unwanted effects are reduced.
- Microspheres reduce dose dumping. Microspheres provide the protection of drugs against environment.
- Microspheres also mask the taste and odor. Microspheres avoids the first pass metabolism.
- Microspheres can be easily injected in body because of their small and spherical size. Microspheres enhance the biological half-life and also improve the bioavailability.

- Controlled release delivery biodegradable microspheres are used to control drug release rates thereby decreasing toxic side effects, and eliminating the inconvenience of repeated injections. Microspheres also reduce the chances of G. I. irritation.
- In case of microspheres, better therapeutic effect for short half-life of drugs can be achieved.
- Microspheres provide freedom from drug and recipients incompatibilities especially with buffer

1.5.4 Limitations:

The costs of the materials and processing of the controlled release preparation, are substantially higher than those of standard formulations. Controlled release rate of microspheres may vary due to certain factors like intrinsic or extrinsic factors may be food, rate of transit through gut, mucin turnover rate etc. The fate of polymer matrix and its effect on the environment. There are differences in release from one to another dosage form. Any loss of integrity in release pattern may cause potential toxicity. The fate of polymer additives such as plasticizers, stabilizers, antioxidants and filers. Reproducibility is less. Low drug loading is done in case of parental microspheres. Process situations like change in temperature, pH, solvent addition, and evaporation/agitation may influence the stability of core particles to be encapsulated. Parental delivery of microspheres may interact or form complex with blood components. The environmental impact of the degradation products of the polymer matrix produced in response to heat, hydrolysis, oxidation, solar radiation or biological agents.

1.5.5 Ideal micro particulate carriers:

The material utilized for the preparation of micro particulates should have the following properties.

- Control of content release
- Increase of therapeutic efficiency
- Protection of drug
- Reduction of toxicity
- Biocompatibility

- Sterilizability
- Relative stability
- Water solubility or dispersibility
- Bio-resorbability
- Target ability
- Polyvalent
- Longer duration of action

The microsphere in pharmaceutical industry for their following applications:

- Masking of taste and odor.
- Delay of volatilization.
- Safe in case of toxic substances.
- Flow of powder is improved.
- Sustained-release, controlled-release, targeted medication can be produced.
- Reduced dose dumping, etc.

1.5.6 Applications of microspheres:

1) Microspheres in vaccine delivery:

The prerequisite of a vaccine is protection against the microorganism or its toxic product. The ideal vaccine must fulfill the requirement of efficacy, safety, convenience in application and cost. The aspect of safety and minimization of adverse reactions a complex issue. The aspect of safety and the degree of the production of antibody responses are closely related to mode of application. Biodegradable delivery systems for vaccines that are given by parenteral route may overcome the shortcoming of the conventional vaccines. The interest in parenteral (subcutaneous, intramuscular, intradermal) carrier lies since they offer specific advantages including the following of the

• Improved antigen city by adjuvant action

• Modulation of antigen release
• Stabilization of antigen.

2)Targeting using micro particulate carriers:

The concept of targeting, i.e. the sites specific drug delivery is a well-established dogma, which is gaining full attention. The therapeutic efficacy of the drug relies on its access and specific interaction with its candidate receptors. The ability to leave the pool in reproducible, efficient and specific manner is enter to drug action mediated by use of a carrier system.

3)Monoclonal antibodies facilitated microspheres targeting:

Monoclonal antibodies targeting microspheres are immune microspheres. This targeting is used to achieve selective targeting to specific sites. Monoclonal antibodies are extremely specific
molecules. This extreme specificity of monoclonal antibodies (Mabs) can be utilized to target microspheres loaded bioactive molecules to selected sites. Mabs can be directly attached to the microsphere by means of covalent coupling. The free aldehyde groups, amino groups or hydroxyl groups on the surface of the microspheres can be linked to the antibodies. ([15,16]).

- Non-specific adsorption and specific adsorption
- Direct coupling
- Coupling via reagent

4)Imaging:

The microspheres have been extensively studied and used for the targeting purposes. Various cells, cell lines, tissues and organs can be imaged using radio labelled microspheres. The particle injected intravenously apart from the portal vein will become entrapped in the capillary bed of the lungs. This phenomenon is abused for the scintigraphic imaging of the tumor masses in lungs using labelled human serum albumin microspheres.

5)Topical porous microspheres:

Micro-sponge are porous microspheres having myriad of interconnected voids of particle size range 5-300μm. Those micro-sponge having capacity to entrap wide range of active ingredients such as emollients, fragrances, essential oils etc., are used as the topical carries system further, these porous microspheres with active ingredients can be incorporated into formulations such as creams, lotions and powders. Micro-sponge consists of non-collapsible structures with porous surface through which active ingredients are released in a controlled manner.

6)Nasal drug delivery:

Intranasal (IN) administration has many theoretical and practical advantages for the local and systemic delivery of a diverse therapeutic compound. IN delivery is needle free, non-invasive, and essentially painless, does not require sterile preparation, and can be self-administered. The large surface area of the nasal mucosa originated from the presence of a large number of microvilli, a porous endothelial membrane, and a highly vascularized epithelium serves a rapid onset of therapeutic effect. It describes various systems, devices, formulations, and methods of delivery of drugs to the nose or nasal cavity. Depending on the therapeutic intent, intranasal drugs may be targeted for local treatment or systematic action. In nasal drug delivery, coupling of bio adhesive properties to microspheres is of great importance because of additional advantages: efficient absorption and enhanced bioavailability of the drug, a much more intimate contact with the mucus layer and reduction in frequency of drug administration due to the reduction in muco-ciliary clearance of drug delivery system adhering to nasal mucosa.

7)Ophthalmic drug delivery:

Polymer exhibits favorable biological behavior such as bio adhesion, permeability-enhancing properties, and interesting physicochemical characteristics, which make it a unique material for the design of ocular drug delivery vehicles. Due to their elastic properties, polymer hydro gels offer better acceptability, with respect to solid or semisolid formulation, for ophthalmic delivery, such as suspensions or ointments, ophthalmic chitosan gels improve adhesion to the mucin, which coats the conjunctiva and the corneal surface of the eye, and increase precorneal drug residence times, showing down drug elimination by the lachrymal flow. In addition, its penetration enhancement has more targeted effect and allows lower doses of the drugs. In contrast, polymer based colloidal system were found to work as transmucosal drug carriers, either facilitating the transport of drugs to the inner eye (chitosan-coated colloidal system containing indomethacin) or their accumulation into the corneal/conjunctival epithelia (chitosan nanoparticulate containing cyclosporine). The micro particulate drug carrier (micro spheres) seems a promising means of topical administration of acyclovir to the eye. The duration of efficacy of the ofloxacin was increased by using high MW (1930 kd) chitosan.

8)Gene delivery:

Gene delivery systems include viral vectors, cationic liposomes, polycation complexes, and microencapsulated systems. Viral vectors are advantageous for gene delivery because they are highly sufficient and have a wide range of cell targets. However, when used in vivo they cause immune responses and oncogenic effects. To overcome the limitations of viral vectors, non-viral delivery systems are considered for gene therapy. Non-viral delivery system has advantages such as ease of preparation, cell/tissue targeting, low immune response, unrestricted plasmid size, and large-scale reproducible production. Polymer has been used as a carrier of DNA for gene delivery applications. Also, polymer could be a useful oral gene carrier because of its adhesive and transport properties in the GI tract. Mac Laughlin et al showed that plasmid DNA containing cytomegalo virus promoter sequence and a luciferase reporter gene could be delivered in vivo by chitosan and depolymerized chitosan oligomers to express a luciferase gene.

9)Intra tumoral and local drug delivery:

Intra- tumoral and local drug delivery strategies have gained momentum recently as a promising modality in cancer therapy. In order to deliver paclitaxel at the tumor site in therapeutically relevant concentration, polymer films were fabricated. Paclitaxel could be loaded at 31% (w/w) in films, which were translucent and flexible. polymer films containing paclitaxel were obtained by casting method with high loading efficiencies and the chemical integrity of molecule was unaltered during preparation according to study.

10)Oral drug delivery:

The potential of polymer films containing diazepam as an oral drug delivery was investigated in rabbits. The results indicated that a film composed of a 1:0.5 drug-polymer mixture might be an effective dosage form that is equivalent to the commercial tablet dosage forms. The ability of polymer to form films may permit its use in the formulation of film dosage forms, as an alternative to pharmaceutical tablets. The pH sensitivity, coupled with the reactivity of the primary amine groups, make polymer a unique polymer for oral drug delivery applications.

11)Buccal drug delivery:

A combination of chitosan membrane and chitosan hydrogel containing lidocaine hydrochloride, a local anesthetic, is a good transparent system for controlled drug delivery and release kinetics Polymer is an excellent polymer to be used for buccal delivery because it has muco/bio adhesive properties and can act as an absorption enhancer. Buccal tablets based on chitosan microspheres containing chlorhexidine diacetate gives prolonged release of the drug in the buccal cavity improving the antimicrobial activity of the drug. The polymer micro particles with no drug incorporated have antimicrobial activity due to the polymer. The buccal bi layered devices (bi laminated films, palavered tablets) using a mixture of drugs (nifedipine and propranolol hydrochloride) and chitosan, with or without anionic crosslinking polymers (polycarbophil, sodium alginate, gellan gum) has promising potential for use in controlled delivery in the oral cavity.

12)Gastrointestinal drug delivery:

Polymer granules having internal cavities prepared by deacidification when added to acidic and neutral media are found buoyant and provided a controlled release of the drug prednisolone. Floating hollow microcapsules of melatonin showed gastro retentive controlled-release delivery system. Release of the drug from these microcapsules is greatly retarded with release lasting for 1.75 to 6.7 hours in simulated gastric fluid. Most of the mucoadhesive microcapsules are retained in the stomach for more than 10 hours e.g., Metoclopramide and glipizide loaded chitosan microspheres.

13)Transdermal drug delivery:

As Polymer has a good film-forming property. The drug release from the devices is affected by the membrane thickness and cross-linking of the film. Chitosan-alginate polyelectrolyte complex has been prepared in-situ in beads and microspheres for potential applications in packaging, controlled release systems and wound dressings. Polymer gel beads are a promising biocompatible and biodegradable vehicle for treatment of local inflammation for drugs like prednisolone which showed sustained release action improving therapeutic efficacy. The rate of drug release was found to be dependent.

14)Colonic drug delivery:

Polymer has been used for the specific delivery of insulin to the colon. The chitosan capsules were coated with enteric coating (Hydroxy propyl methyl cellulose phthalate) and contained, apart from insulin, various additional absorption enhancer and enzyme inhibitor. It was found that capsules specifically disintegrated in the colonic region. It was suggested that this disintegration was due to either the lower pH in the ascending colon as compared to the terminal ileum or to the presence bacterial enzyme, which can degrade the polymer.

15)Multi particulate delivery system:

H. Steckel and F. Mindermann Nogly have prepared chitosan pellets using the extrusion/ spheronisation technology. Microcrystalline cellulose was used as additive in concentrations range from 0-70 %. The powder mixture was extruded using water and dilutes acetic acid in different powder to liquid ratios. The study showed that chitosan pellets with a maximum of 50 % (m/m) could be produced with demineralized water as granulating fluid. The mass fraction of chitosan within in the pallets could be increased to 100% by using dilute acetic acid for the granulation.

Other potential applications include:

Conversion of oil and other liquids to solids for ease of handling

Taste and odor masking

To delay the volatilization

Safe handling of toxic substances.

16)Gastro retentive controlled delivery system:

In which Floating systems are low-density systems that have float over the gastric contents and remain in the stomach for a prolonged period than conventional dosage forms. Gastric emptying of dosage form is extremely variable process and ability to control the emptying time is valuable asset for dosage forms, there are several difficulties are faced in designing controlled released systems for better absorption and enhanced the bioavailability. While the system floats over the gastric contents, the drug is released slowly at the desired rate, which results in increased gastro-retention time and reduces fluctuation in plasma drug concentration. Several polymers are used for gastro retentive controlled delivery system such are Cellulose acetate, Chitosan, Eudragit, Acrycoat, Methocil, Polyacrylates, Polyvinyl acetate, carbopol, Agar, Polyethylene oxide, Polycarbonates, Acrylic resins and Polyethylene oxide etc.

17)Implantable devices:

Microencapsulation has also been used medically for the encapsulation of live cells and vaccines. Biocompatibility can be improved by the encapsulation of artificial cells and biomolecules such as peptides, proteins, and hormones, which can prevent unwanted immunological reactions that would lead to inactivation or rejection. Microspheres are used for isolating materials until their activity is needed. The biotechnology industry employs microspheres to contain organisms and their recombinant products to aid in the isolation of this products.

1.5.7Pharmaceutical Applications:

A number of pharmaceutical microencapsulated products are currently on the market, such as aspirin, theophylline and its derivatives, vitamins, pancreatic lipase, antihypertensives, potassium chloride, progesterone, and contraceptive hormone combinations. Microencapsulated KCL is used to prevent gastrointestinal complications associated with potassium chloride. The dispersibility of the microcapsules and the controlled release of the ions minimize the possibility of local high salt concentrations which could result in ulceration, hemorrhage, or perforation. Microspheres have also found potential applications as injection, or inhalation products. The number of commercially available products does not reflect the amount of research that has been carried out in this area, nor the benefits that can be achieved using this technology. Economic considerations have been a key factor in determining the number of pharmaceutical microencapsulated products. Most encapsulation processes are expensive and require significant capital investment for equipment. An exception is pan or sprays coating and spray drying, since the necessary equipment may already be available within the company. An additional expense is due to the fact of microencapsulation processes.

1.5.8 Types of microspheres:

There are following types of microspheres:

1. Bio-adhesive Microspheres
2. Magnetic Microspheres
    - Therapeutic Microspheres
    - Diagnostic Microspheres
3. Floating Microspheres
4. Polymeric Microspheres
    - Biodegradable Polymeric Microspheres
    - Synthetic Polymeric Microspheres
5. Radioactive Microspheres
6. Mucoadhesive Microspheres

1.5.9 Method of Preparation:

1)Double Emulsion Technique

2)Single Emulsion Technique

3)Coacervation Phase Separation Technique

4)Spray Drying and Spray Congealing Technique

5)Polymerization Technique

- Interfacial Polymerization
- Normal Polymerization
- Suspension Polymerization

6)Solvent Extraction Technique

7)Ionic Gelation Technique

1.5.10 Physicochemical Evaluation:

1) Characterization

2) Particle Size and Shape

3) Electron Spectroscopy for Chemical Analysis

4) Infrared Spectroscopy

5) Density Determination

6) Isoelectric point

7) Angle of Contact

8) Entrapment Efficiency

9) Percentage Yield

10) Swelling Index

11) Invitro Methods:

    a) Beaker Method

    b) Interface Diffusion Method

    c) Modified Keshary Chein Cell

12) In vivo Methods:

    a) Animal Models

    b) Buccal Absorption Test

13) In Vitro In Vivo Correlation:

    a) Percent of Drug Dissolved In Vitro Vs Peak Plasma Concentration

    b) Percent of Drug Dissolved Vs Percent of Drug Absorbed

c) Dissolution Rate Vs Absorption Rate

d) Percent of Drug Dissolved Vs Serum Drug Concentration

e) Percent of Drug Dissolved Vs Percent of the Dose Excreted in urine

1.5.11 Recent advancement in microsphere:

Important utilization of chitosan polymer cholesterol – lowering effects

- Increase stability of drug
- Orthopedic patients
- Cosmetics industry
- Dental medicine
- Wound healing properties
- Chitosan as Permeation enhancer
- Chitosan as Mucoadhesive Excipient
- Effect of Chitosan: citric acid ratio on drug release
- Chitosan as Permeation Enhancer.

2. LITERATURE REVIEW

- Kaustubh V. Gavali, et al., (2019), Asian Journal of Pharmaceutical and Research, Vol. 9, Issue 2, April-June 2019, emphasized that microspheres are multi particulate drug delivery system which are prepared to obtain prolonged or controlled drug delivery to improve bioavailability, stability and to target the drug to specific site at a predetermined rate. They are made from polymeric waxy or other protective materials such as natural, semi synthetic and synthetic polymers. The range of techniques for the preparation of microspheres provides multiple options to control as drug administration aspects and to enhance the therapeutic efficacy of a given drug. These delivery systems offer maximum advantages over conventional dosage forms, which accounts for improved efficacy, reduced toxicity, improved patient compliance and convenience, reduced dosage frequency.
- Bindu Madhavi, et al., (2011), Journal for Drugs and Medicines, Vol. 3, Issue 1, April 2011, reported that Venlafaxine hydrochloride is the free soluble with antidepressant activity. Being highly soluble drug there is possibility of burst effects. To reduce the adverse effects due to burst effect and to have the sustain action of the drug we have prepared the ethyl cellulose microspheres of the drug. The microspheres were prepared by the emulsification and solvent evaporation method. The drug release was found to be sustained for 16hrs and was found to follow the Peppas kinetics.
- Kulkarni Giriraj T, et al., (2011), Journal of Chronotherapy and Drug Delivery, Vol 2, Issue 3, 2011:113-119, studied that plant- based drugs are used by the human race since times immemorial for different ailments. But, these phytomedicines suffer limitations, which are mainly due to stability issues and poor lipid solubility. To overcome these problems, novel drug delivery systems are being developed for phytomedicines. These herbal novel drug delivery systems include vesicular delivery systems such as liposomes, phytosomes, ethosomes, transferosomes, particulate delivery systems such as microspheres, micro pellets, nanoparticles, and micro and nano emulsions. Many herbal drugs have been incorporated into these systems for improvement of stability, bioavailability and reduction of toxicity.
- Barish, et al., (2010), studied that developed oral sustained release microspheres of Cefazolin sodium to attain prolonged action, which can reduce its side effects and provide more safety and efficacy. The microspheres were formulated by solvent evaporation

method using the polymer Guar gum. Five formulations were prepared with 1:1, 1:2, 1:3, 1:4. 1:5 drug: polymer ratio. They were comparatively evaluated for their better release profile.

- Manoj Kumar Das, et al., (2019), International Journal of Current Pharmaceutical Research, Vol 11, Issue 4, 2019, carried out a study that the targeted drug delivery is designed for endeavoring to concentrate the drug in the tissues of curiosity while reducing relative concentration of medication in the remaining tissues. The surrounding tissues are not affected by the drug. Controlled drug delivery system can overcome the problems of conventional drug therapy and gives better therapeutic efficacy of a drug. There are various approaches in delivering a therapeutic substance to the target site in a sustained controlled release fashion. In future various other strategies, microspheres will find the central place in novel drug delivery, particularly in diseased cell sorting, diagnostics, gene and genetic materials, safe, targeted and effective in vivo delivery and supplements as miniature versions of diseased organ and tissues in the body.
- Sachin R. Patel, et al., (2014), An International Journal of Pharmaceutical Sciences, Vol. 5, Issue 1, Jan- Mar 2014, aimed to formulate and evaluate floating microspheres of highly water- soluble drugs Venlafaxine hydrochloride, using cellulose acetate. The microspheres were prepared by solvent evaporation method. Release studies showed that microspheres that able to release the drug in sustain manner. Selected formulations were subjected to kinetic studies and stability studies. The range of techniques for the preparation of microspheres provides multiple options to control as drug administration aspects and to enhance the therapeutic efficacy.
- Priya Shukla, et al., (2015), International Journal of Pharmacy and Analytical Research, Vol 4, Issue 3, Jul- Sep 2015, the range of Techniques for the preparation of microspheres offers a Variety of opportunities to control aspects of drug administration and enhance the therapeutic efficacy of a given drug. There are various approaches in delivering a therapeutic substance to the target site in a sustained controlled release fashion. One such approach is using microspheres as carriers for drugs also known as microparticles. It is the reliable means to deliver the drug to the target site with specificity and to maintain the desired concentration at the site of interest. Microspheres received much attention not only for prolonged release, but also for targeting of anticancer drugs.
- Dipak A. Patil, et al., (2019), World Journal of Pharmacy and Pharmaceutical Sciences, Vol 8, Issue 3, 2019, developed that microspheres are ball bearing effects because of their spherical shape. The therapeutic efficacy of microspheres contain drug depends upon their

characteristics that can be altered in required terms by altering materials, methods, polymers or techniques used. A Microspheres has its drug dispersed throughout the particle i.e. the internal structure is a matrix of drug and polymeric excipients. It is the reliable means to deliver the drug to the target site with specificity, if modified, and to maintain the desired concentration at the site of interest without untoward effects. Microspheres received much attention not only for prolonged release, but also for targeting of anticancer drugs to the tumor.

- Kausalya Arumugam, et al., (2021), International Journal of Pharmacy and Pharmaceutical Sciences, Vol. 13, Issue 7, 2021, focused that the microspheres were formulated by the solvent evaporation method using different ratios of polymers like Carbopol 940, ethyl cellulose, hydroxy propyl methyl cellulose K4M. The particle size ranged from 258.1±2.21µm to 278±2.86µm. The IR spectrum revealed that there was no interaction between the drug and polymer. Ciprofloxacin microspheres showed the good flowing property.
- Srinivas Thota, et al., (2021), International Journal of Research in Pharmaceutical Sciences and Technology, Vol. 2, Issue 4, 2021, pertained that Diclofenac sodium undergoes extensive first pass metabolism. The ethyl cellulose based sustained release diclofenac sodium microsphere is to reduce the dosing frequency to achieve targeted drug delivery system. The diclofenac sodium loaded ethyl cellulose microspheres were formulated by emulsification technique and the physicochemical properties of the formulations were characterized. The percentage drug content was studied in three different pH media (pH 1.2, pH 6.8 and pH 8.0).
- Vikrant K. Nikam, et al., (2012), International Journal of Pharmaceutical and Chemical Sciences, Vol 1, Issue 1, Mar 2012, designed and developed that microspheres are well designed controlled drug delivery system can overcome some of the problems of conventional therapy and enhance the therapeutic efficacy of a given drug. A Microspheres has its drug dispersed throughout the particle i.e. the internal structure is a matrix of drug and polymeric excipients It is the reliable means to deliver the drug to the target site with specificity, if modified, and to maintain the desired concentration at the site of interest without untoward effects. Microsphere received much attention not only for prolonged release, but also for targeting of anticancer drugs to the tumor. Microsphere are spherical microparticles, and are used where consistent and predictable particle surface area is important.

- Anam Abrar, et al., (2020), International Journal of Health Sciences, Vol. 1, Issue 2, 2020 Mar- Apr, aimed that this study was undertaken to evaluate the formulation of the microspheres for antiulcer drug using natural polymer Acacia nilotica gum. It is widely used in various ayurvedic formulations and it is used for various ailments such as cancer, cold, cough, diarrhea, dysentery, fever, hypertension, ophthalmic, tuberculosis, smallpox. It is used to formulate microspheres for antiulcer drugs.
- Chandrawanshi Mayuri J, et al., (2018), International Journal of Pharmacy and Pharmaceutical Research, Vol 12, Issue 4, July 2018, carried out a study that microspheres designed to overcome some of the problems of conventional therapy and enhance the therapeutic efficacy of a given drug. To get the desired effect the drug should deliver at the target tissue in an optimal amount in the right period of time with maximum therapeutic effect and minimum side effect. Microspheres are evaluated by methods like Physicochemical Evaluation Characterization, Particle size, and shape, Electron spectroscopy for chemical analysis, In vitro methods, In vitro-In vivo correlations, Swelling Index etc.
- Sarlesh Rajput, et al., (2012), World Journal of Pharmacy and Pharmaceutical Sciences,Vol 1, Issue 1, 422-438, 2012, formulated and studied the concept of targeted drug delivery is designed for attempting to concentrate the drug in the tissues of interest while reducing the relative concentration of the medication in the remaining tissues. As a result, drug is localized on the targeted site. Hence, surrounding tissues are not affected by the drug. So, carrier technology offers an intelligent approach for drug delivery by coupling the drug to a carrier particle such as microspheres, nanoparticles, liposomes, niosomes, etc., which modulates the release and absorption characteristics of the drug. It is the reliable means to deliver the drug to the target site with specificity, if modified, and to maintain the desired concentration at the site of interest without untoward effects.
- B. Meenashree, et al., (2014), International Journal of Pharmaceutical Science and Research, Vol 3, Issue 5, 2014, pertained that Musa acuminata, commonly known as banana plant is vastly being consumed across the world. It is known for many pharmacological activities and reports show that phenolic compounds mainly contribute to this trait. In the present investigation, quantitative analysis of phenolic compound was carried out on ethanol (96%), acetone and petroleum ether extracts of fresh banana leaf by modified Folin- Ciocalteu method. Total phenolic recovery was found to be maximum in petroleum ether followed by acetone and ethanol. This study showed that Musa acuminata leaf is a good source of phenolic compounds. In addition, the leaf extracts were tested for

antimicrobial activities. All the three extracts showed excellent antifungal activities against two pathogenic fungi, but failed to show any antibacterial activities.

- Harsh Bansal, et al., (2011), International Journal of Pharmaceutical Sciences, Vol 10, Issue 1, September- October 2011, emphasized that A well designed controlled drug delivery system can overcome the problems of convention drug therapy and gives better therapeutic efficacy of a drug. Microsphere are also undersigned as novel/controlled drug delivery system having particle size less than 200μm. The therapeutic efficacy of microspheres containing drug depends upon their characteristics that can be altered in required terms by altering materials, methods, polymers or techniques used. With emphasis on preparation, application, biocompatible and their stability to obtain the required or enhanced therapeutic efficacy of a given drug, it become necessary to deliver that particular agent to the target tissues in optimal amount at right period of time with minimum toxicity/side effect.
- Kanav Midha, et al., (2015), International Journal of Recent Scientific Research, Vol. 6, Issue, 8, pp.5859-5867, August, 2015, carried out a study that microspheres are well designed controlled drug delivery system can overcome some of the problems of conventional therapy. There are various approaches in delivering a therapeutic substance to the target site in a sustained controlled release. Among them microsphere drug delivery system has gained enormous attention due to its wide range of application as it covers targeting the drug to particular site to imaging and helping the diagnostic features. Microspheres received much attention not only for prolonged release, but also for targeting of anticancer drugs to the tumor. The purpose is to compile various types of microspheres, different methods to preparation, its applications and various parameters to evaluate their efficiency.
- Anuj Malik, et al., (2017), International Journal of Scientific Research, Vol. 6, Issue 3, March 2017, focused on a study that microspheres are particulate drug delivery systems which are prepared to obtain prolonged or controlled drug delivery. These delivery systems offer maximum advantages over conventional dosage forms, which accounts for improved efficacy, reduced toxicity, improved patient compliance and convenience, reduced dosage frequency. Microspheres are like Floating microspheres, Bio adhesive microspheres, Polymeric microspheres, Biodegradable polymeric microspheres, Magnetic microspheres, Radioactive microspheres, Synthetic polymeric microspheres and are prepared by methods like Spray Drying, Solvent Evaporation, Single emulsion technique, Double emulsion

technique, Phase separation co-acervation technique, Spray drying and spray congealing, Quassi emulsion solvent, diffusion Solvent extraction.

- Dhadde Gurunath S, et al., (2021), Asian Journal of Pharmacy and Technology, Vol. 11, Issue 2, 2021, aimed to carry out a study that microspheres are one of the novel drug delivery system in which effective therapeutic alternative to conventional or immediate release single-unit dosage forms. Microspheres can be characterized as solid, diameter having between 1-1000μm. There are different types of microspheres. These microspheres prepared and fill them in a hard gelatin or compress them directly. The microspheres which are prepared by using different technique that are changes their effectiveness and administration of the dosage form as compare to conventional dosage form. Microsphere will be evaluated by using different methods that analyses quality of the microsphere.

3. AIM AND OBJECTIVE

AIM:

This Research work aims to formulate and evaluate microspheres of Musa Paradisiaca so as to study the targeted as well as prolonged drug release in the diseased area, to overcome the limitations of conventional dosage forms and to increase bioavailability.

OBJECTIVE:

- To convert the herbal extract into a novel dosage form.
- The objective of the present study was to microencapsulate the Musa paradisiaca extract for sustained release or prolonged drug release.
- To increase the shelf life of the drug by microsphere drug delivery system.
- To provide constant and prolonged therapeutic effect.
- Reduces the dosing frequency fluctuation in therapeutic blood level is avoided.
- Improves patient compliance.
- To increase the t1/2 as well as shelf life of the drug and to reduce the dose.
- To overcome the limitations of conventional dosage forms.
- To increase bioavailability.

4.PLAN OF WORK

In order to meet the aims and objectives, the present work was planned in the following manner.

- Authentication for the selected plant.
- Procurement of dried powder of Musa Paradisiaca leaves.
- Selection of polymers.
- Selection of microencapsulating carrier.
- Pre formulation studies.
- Phytochemical Evaluations:
    - Total phenol content
    - Flavonoid content
- Qualitative and Quantitative analysis.
- Compatibility study – Fourier Transform Infrared Spectroscopy (FTIR).
- Formulation of microspheres from the Musa Paradisiaca leaves using ethyl cellulose carrier (extract: polymers in different ratio) by Solvent Extraction Technique.
- Evaluation:
    - Particle size and shape
    - Percentage yield
    - Drug entrapment efficiency
    - Scanning electron microscope study
    - FTIR spectra analysis
    - Bulk density
    - Tapped density
    - Swelling index
    - Angle of repose
    - % Compressibility index
- Standard curve of synthetic drug.
- Study of the invitro release pattern of drug from ethyl cellulose microspheres containing Musa Paradisiaca leaf extract.
- Stability studies of ethyl cellulose microspheres containing Musa Paradisiaca leaf extract.

5. PLANT PROFILE

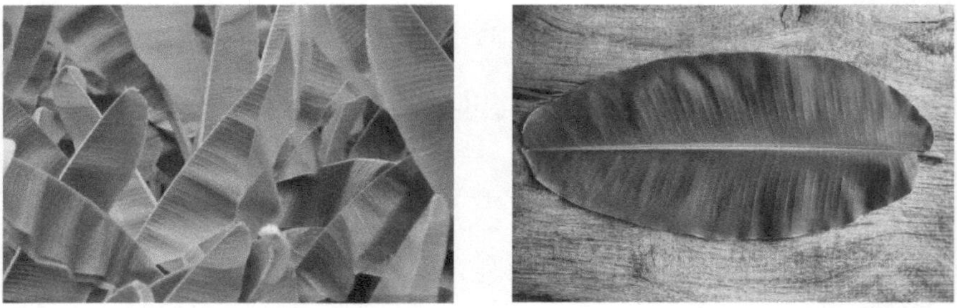

Fig 1: Musa paradisiaca leaves

5.1 Scientific Classification:

Kingdom	:	Plantae
Subkingdom	:	Tracheobionta
Super division	:	Spermatophyta
Division	:	Magnoliophyta
Class	:	Liliopsida
Subclass	:	Zingiberidae
Order	:	Zingiberales
Family	:	Musaceae
Genus	:	Musa L.
Species	:	M. paradisiacal L.

5.2 Description:

Color : Lime, olive green, to dark green.

Banana leaves are large, wide, elongated, and slightly rounded, averaging two meters in length, a half a meter in width, and 8 – 12 leaves per tree. The surface of those leaves will be waxy, flexible, and glossy.

5.3 Synonyms : Banana tree, Plantain tree, Plantain, Banana.

5.4 Medicinal uses : The leaves are used by the tribal in Western Ghats in India for bandaging cuts, blisters and ulcers. The leaves have been shown to possess ulcer healing activity. The flower, stem and the juice of green banana leaves are equally useful. Banana plant and banana leaves are not only food for elephant and other animals but also are of incredible medicinal value for human being. Banana leaves, at their tender stage, can be used to make poultice for treating burns and astringent ashes of unripe peel and leaves are effective for preventing the growth of malignant ulcers and are suitable to treat diarrhea and dysentery. The juice of banana leaf is useful in case of cough, cold, breathing problem, dropsy constipation, dysentery, acidity, high BP, blood disorder or poisoning and also for liver problem. The consumption of half cup of the juice of green leaf every morning, without use of sweetener or salt, will prevent various diseases (i.e. Bronchitis, Nephritis, T.B, pleurisy). It purifies blood and is used as topical for chest pains. The chlorophyll in banana leaves protect us from intestinal ulcer, leukemia and skin diseases. An infusion of the banana leaf, combined with sugarcane roots, is used to hasten childbirth. The Leaves are applied as a vesicant on blistering. It is tied onto the forehead to relieve a headache. The large leaves are used as a plate for eating foods. The leaf sheath is used as a temporary binding.

5.5 Pharmacological activities:

1) Antioxidant activity

2) Anticancer effect

12) Antidiarrheal

13) Antiallergic

3) Antiulcer activity

4) Antidiabetic effect

5) Antimicrobial activity

6) Wound healing attribute

7) Effect on atherosclerosis

8) Anti angiogenic activity

9) Antilithiatic

10) Analgesic

11) Antihypertensive

14) Diuretic

15) Hypolipidemic

16) Hypoglycemic

17) Hair growth promoting

18) Hemostatic

19) Muscle relaxant

20) Mutagenic

21) Vasodilatory activities

22) Anti-snake venom activity

5.6 Anti- diabetic activities of Musa paradisiaca:

Detailed studies in pharmacological investigations revealed that Musa paradisiaca leaves are screened for antidiabetic activity. Various ingredients have been identified from different parts of Musa paradisiaca and include serotonin, dopamine, flavonoids, quercetin, 3- O-galactoside, leucocyanidin, 3-O-glucoside, 3-0-rhamnosyl glucoside, and acyl steryl glycosides. Acyl steryl glycoside such as sitoindoside-I, sitoindoside-II, sitoindoside-III, sitoindoside-IV and steryl glycosides have also been isolated. To investigate the antidiabetic activity of Musa paradisiaca, different parts of the plants such as leaves, peels, roots, stems were collected. The ethanolic extracts and the hexane and chloroform fraction of leaves showed promising antidiabetic activity. Further the isolated compounds from the active fractions did not show the antidiabetic activity. The leaves demonstrated lowering blood glucose level at 500mg/kg body weight.

5.7 Chemical constituents of Musa paradisiaca:

Different chemical constituents like

- Apigenin glycoside
- Myricetin glycoside

- Myricetin – 3- O – rutinoside
- Nanringenin glycoside
- Kaempferol – 3 – O – rutinoside
- Dopamine
- N – acetyl serotonin
- Rutin

have been reported in different parts and varieties of banana.

Structure of the major active constituents in Musa paradisiaca leaves:

Apigenin glycosides

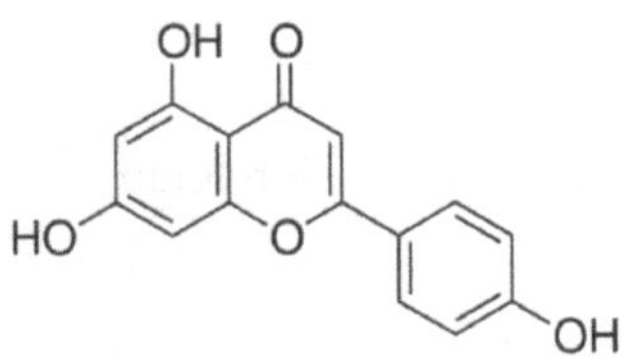

Fig: 2

Myricetin glycoside

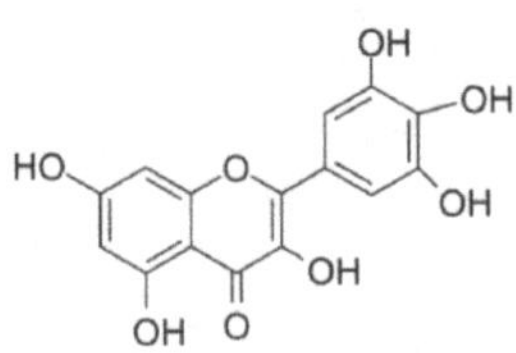

Fig: 3

Myricetin-3-O-rutinoside Kaempferol-3-O-

rutinoside

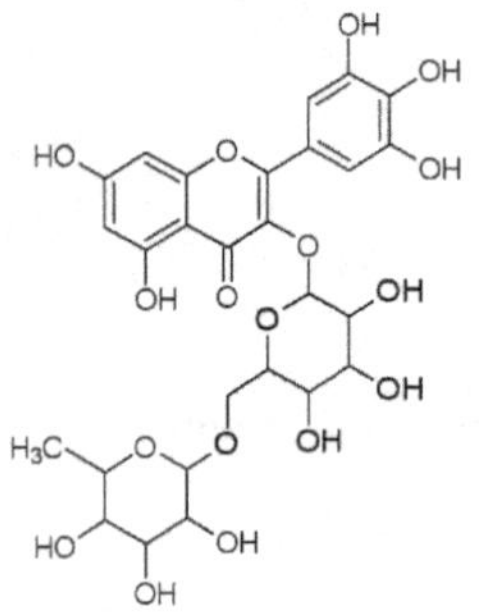

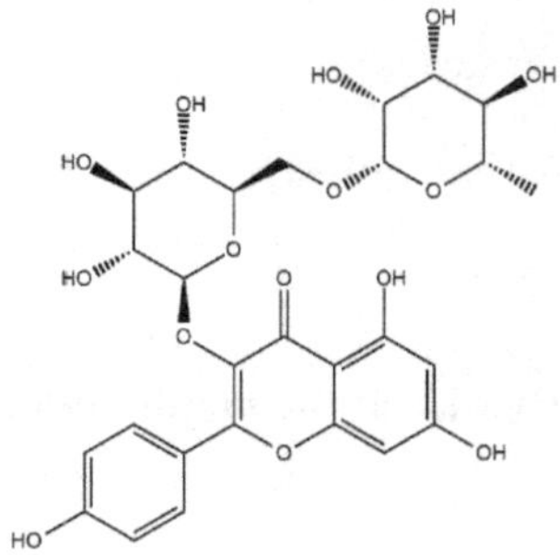

Fig: 4 **Fig: 5**

Dopamine N- acetyl serotonin

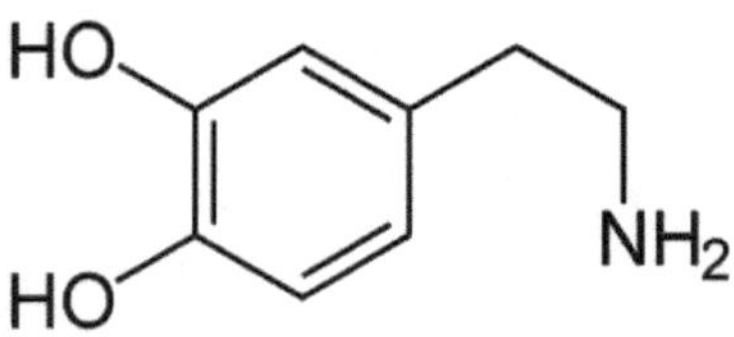

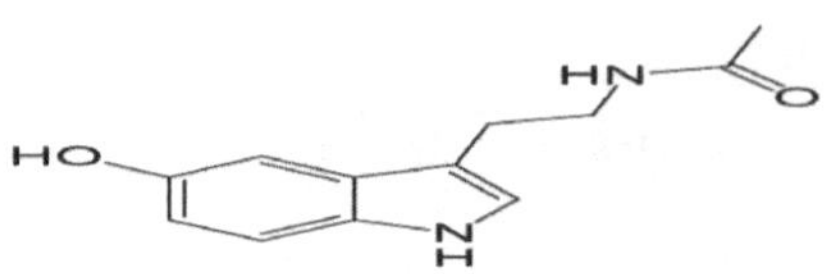

Fig: 6 **Fig: 7**

Rutin

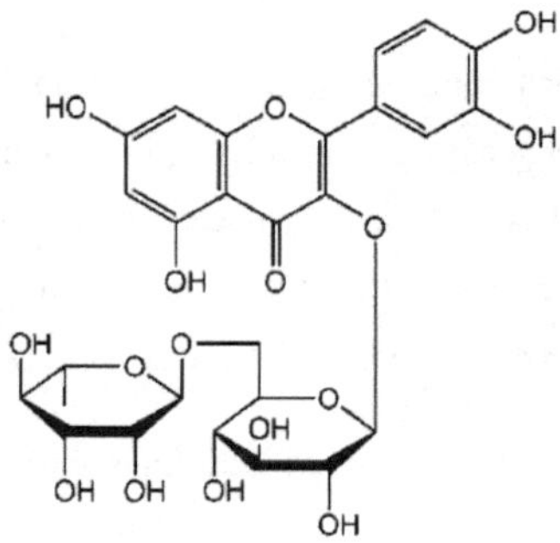

Fig: 8

6. EXCIPIENTS PROFILE

6.1 ETHYL CELLULOSE:

Ethyl cellulose is a derivative of cellulose in which some of the hydroxyl groups on the repeating glucose units are converted into ethyl ether groups. It is mainly used as a thin – film coating material for coating paper, vitamin and medical pills, and for thickeners in cosmetics and in industrial processes. Ethyl cellulose is also used as a food additive as an emulsifier. Food grade ethyl cellulose is one of few non – toxic films and thickeners which are not water soluble.

- **Synonyms** : Ethyl cellulose, Aquacoat, Ethocel, Surelease, Cellulose ethyl ether, Ethocel MED, EC, Ethyl cellulose (fr), Etil cellulose(It), Etilcelulose(Port).
- **Chemical name CAS registry number :** Cellulose ethyl ether [9004-57-3]
- **Empirical formula** : $C_{20}H_{38}O_{11}$
- **Molecular weight** : 454.5
- **Structural formula:**

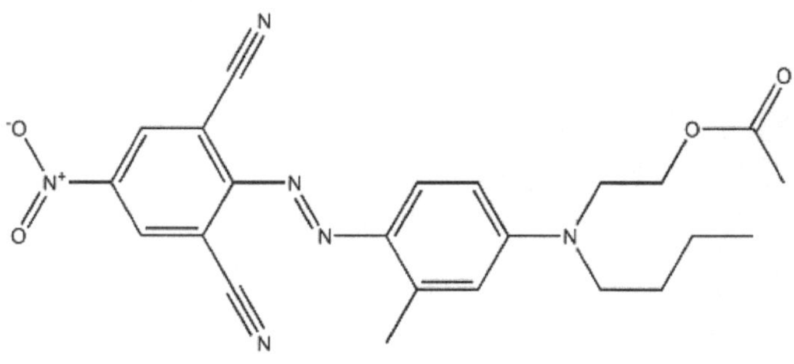

Fig 9: Structure of Ethyl Cellulose

- **Description** : A thermoplastic, colorless powder composed of an ethyl ether of cellulose. Commercial ethyl cellulose (EC) has an ethoxy content of 43-50%. It softens at about 100-140C and is compatible with resins, waxes, oils and plasticizers. Ethyl cellulose forms a tough, flexible, transparent film that is very wear resistant. It is used in food containers; hot melt adhesives, inks and as protective coatings for paper and textiles. Ethyl cellulose is rarely used in conservation because it oxidizes readily and is thermally unstable.

- **Functional category** : Coating agent, flavoring fixative, tablet binder, tablet filler, viscosity increasing agent, fill former, drug carrier, or stabilizer.

- **Typical properties:**

- Density : $0.4 gm/cm^3$
- Glass transition temperature : 129-133C
- Solubility : Ethyl cellulose is practically insoluble in glycerin, propylene glycol, and water. Ethyl cellulose that contains less than 46.5% of ethoxy group is freely soluble in chloroform, methyl acetate, and tetrahydrofuran, and in mixtures of aromatic hydrocarbons with ethanol (95%). Ethyl cellulose that contains not less than 46.5% of ethoxy groups is freely soluble in chloroform, ethanol (95%), ethyl acetate, methanol, and toluene.
- Specific gravity : $1.12- 1.15 g/cm^3$.

6.1.1Applications in Pharmaceutical Technology:

- It is used in bio-adhesive and mucoadhesive drug delivery systems.
- It is used in pharmaceutical coating processes.
- It is used in extended release (ER) solid dosage forms.
    - In coated extended release formulations.

    - In extended release polymeric matrices.
- It is used in osmotic drug delivery systems.
    - In SPM formulation of osmotic system.
    - In central core of osmotic systems
- It is used in enteric coated solid dosage forms.
- It is used as compressibility enhancers.
- It is used as thickening and stabilizing agents.
- It is used as fillers in solid dosage forms.
- It is used as binders in granulation process.
- It is used as disintegrating agents.
- It is used as taste masking agents.

6.2 DICHLOROMETHANE:

Dichloromethane is an organo chloride compound with the formula CH_2CL_2. DCM's volatility and ability to dissolve a wide range of organic compounds make it a useful solvent for many chemical processes. In the food industry, it is used to decaffeinate coffee and tea as well as to prepare extracts of hops and other flavorings. Its volatility has led to its use as an aerosol spray propellant and as a blowing agent for polyurethane foams.

- **Synonyms** : Methylene chloride, Methane dichloride, Solaesthin, Solmethin, Dichlormethane, Chlorure de methylene, Freon 30, Metylenu chlorek, Metaclen.

- **Chemical name CAS registry number** : Methylene chloride [75 – 09 – 2]

- **Empirical formula** : CH_2CL_2

- **Molecular weight** : 84.93g.mol^{-1}

- **Structural formula:**

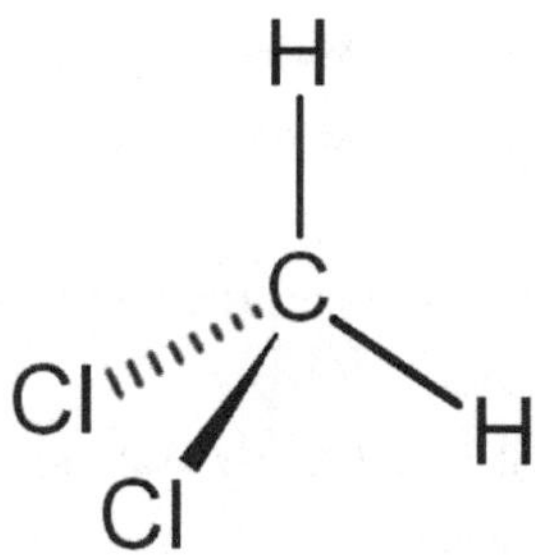

Fig 10: Structure of Dichloromethane

- **Description** : Dichloromethane appears as a clear, dense, non – flammable colorless, volatile liquid chlorinated hydrocarbon with a sweet, penetrating, ether – like odor. Non-combustible by if exposed to high temperatures may emit toxic chloride fumes. Vapors are narcotic in high concentrations. Colorless liquid with a chloroform – like odor. Used as a solvent and paint remover. It is a member of chloromethanes and a volatile organic compound.

- **Functional category** : Solvent, paint remover, polar aprotic solvent, carcinogenic agent, refrigerant, aerosol spray propellant, blowing agent.

- **Typical properties:**
  - Density : 1.3266g/cm

- Solubility : Miscible in ethyl acetate, alcohol, hexanes, benzene, CCl_4, diethyl ether, $CHCl_3$. It is moderately soluble in water and soluble in most organic solvents such as ethanol, ether, phenols, aldehydes and ketones. Its evaporation rate is 27.5. DCM vapors are heavier than air.

6.2.1 Applications in pharmaceutical technology:

- It is used as a solvent in the pharmaceutical and chemical industry for chemical reactions, purification and isolation of intermediates or products.
- It is used as a blowing agent in foam blowing, for plastics processing.
- It is used as an extraction solvent in the food industry, in metal cleaning, in paint and varnish removers.
- It is used in aerosol formulations, in paints, sealants and adhesives.
- It is used as a laboratory chemical.
- It is used as a heat transfer fluid and for removal of photo resistant coatings in the production of printed circuit boards.
- It is used by the pharmaceutical industry as a process solvent in the manufacture of steroids, antibiotics, vitamins, and to a lesser extent as a solvent in the coating of tablets.
- It is used in aerosols as a strong solvent, flammability suppressant, vapor pressure depressant and viscosity thinner.

6.3 GELATIN

Gelatin is an animal protein made by boiling the collagenous material from animal bones, hides, and skins. Pig and cattle bones are typically used to make gelatin. Gelatin has many uses, including use in cooking, industrial uses, cosmetics and photography. It consists of eighteen amino acids, eight of which are considered essential. It is brittle when dry and rubbery when moist. Gelatin is generally recognized as safe by the FDA. Gelatin derived from pig skin is normally referred to as type A gelatin and gelatin derived from beef skin is referred to as type B gelatin. Gel strength and viscosity are the most important physical properties of gelatin.

❖ **Synonym**: Teleostean gelatin, prionex (R), gelatin, gel foam, gelatin foam, gal foam, pharma-gel.

❖ **Chemical name CAS registry number**: Gelatin [9000 – 70 – 8]

❖ **Empirical formula**: $C_6H_{12}O_6$

❖ **Molecular weight**: 15 to 400kDa

❖ **Structure:**

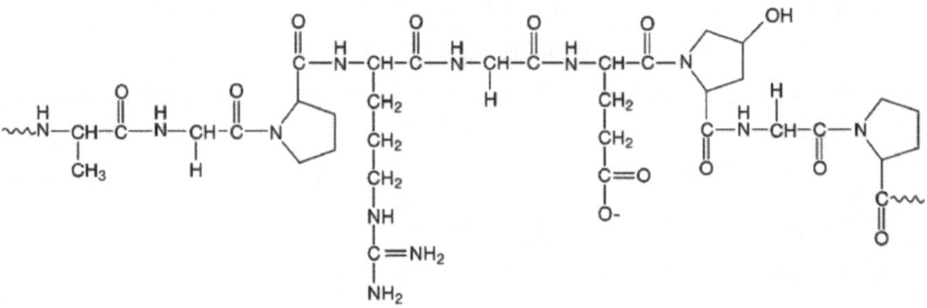

Fig 11: Structure of gelatin

❖ **Description:** Gelatin is a tasteless and odorless taste. It is a somewhat transparent, brittle solid, pale yellow to beige in color and it can come as sheets, flakes, or as a powder. It contains about 10% moisture and is hygroscopic. Gelatin has a long history of safe use in a wide range of biomedical and pharmaceutical applications.

❖ **Functional category:** Thickening agent, gelling agent in food, beverages, medications, drug and vitamin capsules, photographic films and papers, and cosmetics.

❖ **Typical properties:**

- Density: 1.2
- Solubility: Below 3540C gelatin swells and absorbs approximately 5 to 10 times its weight of water to form a gel. Gelatin is soluble in polar solvents like

glycerol and acetic acid, more soluble in hot than in cold water, and insoluble in organic solvents like alcohol.

- Specific gravity:1.01

6.3.1Applications in pharmaceutical technology:

- It is used as a binder in tablets and acts as a matrix in vitamin coating.
- Low endotoxin gelatins are the basis for plasma expanders, vaccines and hemostatic sponges.
- It is used to enhance the remaining circulating blood in emergency situations.
- It is used as an excipient in the production of hard capsules and soft gels.
- It is used as a stabilizer in some vaccines.
- It is used as an emulsifier and extender in the production of reduced fat margarine products.
- It is used for the fabrication of particulate drug delivery systems because of its biocompatible and biodegradable nature.
- It is used in the manufacture of suppositories, surgical sponges and bacterial growth media.
- It is used in the food industry as a thickening agent.

7. MATERIALS AND METHODS

7.1 MATERIALS:

Table 1: List of Reagents and Chemicals

Materials	Sources
Musa paradisiaca leaves	Herbal plant and powder shop, Coimbatore.
Ethyl cellulose	Himedia laboratories Ltd. Mumbai, 400086.
Dichloro methane	Loba chemicals, Mumbai.
Bromophenol red	Loba chemicals, Mumbai.
Gelatin	Loba chemicals, Mumbai.
Potassium dihydrogen phosphate	Nice chemicals.
Sodium hydroxide	Fine chem.., Ltd.

Table 2: List of Equipment

Name of Equipment	Name of Manufacturer
FT - IR	Schimadzu
Scanning Electron Microscope	Hitachi S - 450
UV – Visible spectrophotometer Double beam	Schimadzu Pharmaspec 1700
Single Pan Digital Balance	Afcoset
Mechanical stirrer	Electrocrafts Pvt. Ltd. Mumbai
Dissolution apparatus USP XXIII	Electro lab, Mumbai
Microscope	Unilab
Digital pH meter	Hanna Instruments

7.2 METHODS:

7.2.1 Authentication for the selected plant:

The leaves of Musa paradisiaca were collected from the local areas of Coimbatore, Tamil Nadu, India. The collected leaves were authenticated by Botanical Survey of India (BSI), Coimbatore.

7.2.2 Procurement of dried powder of Musa paradisiaca leaves:

The leaves of Musa paradisiaca were collected from the nearby areas of Coimbatore, Tamil Nadu. And the leaves were cleaned and shade dried at room temperature.

7.2.3 Selection of polymers:

7.2.3.1 Ethyl Cellulose:

Ethyl cellulose is the most commonly used polymer for sustained release, but it is also used for moisture protection and taste masking. It is made by chemical substitution of the naturally occurring polymer, cellulose. It is insoluble, but permeable in water and guarantees pH independent drug release. Ethyl cellulose is insoluble in water and soluble in organic solvents. This polymer has excellent strength at room temperature but its strength decreases rapidly with increasing temperature. Ethyl cellulose finds uses in food packaging applications and as a barrier coating for controlled drug release of pharmaceutical products. It is made by chemical substitution of the naturally occurring polymer, cellulose.

7.2.4 Selection of microencapsulating carrier:

7.2.4.1 Dichloromethane:

Dichloromethane acts as a solvent. It appears as a colorless liquid with a sweet, penetrating, ether like odor. It has a role as a polar aprotic solvent. It is primarily used as a solvent in paint removers, but is also used in aerosol formulations, as a solvent in the manufacture of pharmaceuticals, as a degreasing agent. It is a highly volatile liquid, but it is neither flammable nor explosive in air.

7.2.4.2 Gelatin:

Gelatin is a translucent, colorless, flavorless food ingredient, commonly derived from collagen taken from animal body parts. It is brittle when dry and rubbery when moist. It is commonly used as gelling agent in food, beverages, medications, drug and vitamin capsules, photographic films and papers, and cosmetics. Substances containing gelatin or functioning in a similar way are called gelatinous substances. Gelatin is an irreversibly hydrolyzed form of collagen wherein the hydrolysis reduces protein fibrils into smaller peptides; depending on the physical and chemical methods of denaturation.

7.2.5 Pre-formulation studies:

7.2.5.1 Physicochemical parameters:

1. Organoleptic properties:

2. Bulk characterization studies:

a) Crystallinity and polymorphism
b) Hygroscopicity
c) Fine particle characterization
d) Bulk density
e) Powder flow properties
f) Compression properties
g) Physical description

3. Solubility analysis:

a) Intrinsic solubility determination
b) pKa determination
c) Partition coefficient
d) Dissolution studies
e) Common ion effect

4. Stability analysis:

a) In toxicology formulations
c) Solid state stability

b) Solution stability

1.Organoleptic properties:

Color: It should be Unappealing to the eye and determined by either instrumental methods or visible method that varies from batch to batch. Coating of body in variable color can be done if found undesirable. Odor and taste: For unpalatable drug use of less soluble chemical form or suppress it by flavors, excipients, coating etc. Drug substances which irritating to skin should be handle with precautions. Flavors, dyes, excipients used will affect stability and bioavailability. Color may be off-white, cream yellow, tan, shiny. Odor may be pungent, sulfurous, fruity, aromatic and odorless. Taste may be acidic, bitter, bland, intense, sweet and tasteless.

2.Bulk characterization studies:

It is needed to identify all the solid forms that may exist as a consequence of the synthetic stage such as the presence of polymorphs. Bulks properties such as particle size, bulk density, surface morphology may be changed during the development process and to avoid mislead predictions of solubility and stability which depends on a particular crystalline form. Bulk characterizations:

a) Crystallinity and polymorphism:

The structure of a solid compound refers as crystallinity and these structures disappear in the liquid and vapor states. It can be classified as Internal structures (cubic, tetragonal, hexagonal, rhombic, etc.), Solid habits (platy, needle, tabular, prismatic, bladed, etc.), Changing the internal structures alter the crystal habits, Changing the chemical form (e.g. salt formation) alter both the internal structure and crystal habit. Polymorphism is the ability of the compound to crystallize as more than one distinct crystalline of the same compounds. They have different physicochemical properties (melting point, density, vapor pressure, X-ray, color, crystal shape, hardness, solubility, dissolution rate and bioavailability). During pre-formulation, it is important to identify the polymorph that is stable at room temperature.

b) Hygroscopicity:

Hygroscopic (a substance that exist in a dynamic equilibrium with water). This process depends on the relative humidity of the surroundings. It is characterized by Karl fisher, gravimetric, TGA, or Gas chromatography methods. It is significances as changes in moisture content that affects stability, flowability, compatibility, etc.

c) Fine particle characterization:

Certain physical and chemical properties of drug substances are affected by the particle size distribution, including drug dissolution rate, bioavailability, content uniformity, taste, texture color, and stability. Methods of evaluation of particle size and distribution includes light microscope with a calibrated grid, Sedimentation techniques, Stream scanning, Coulter counter and Surface area determination by BET nitrogen adsorption method.

c)Bulk density:

Bulk density of a compound varies substantially with the method of crystallization, milling or formulation once a density problem is identified it is often easily corrected by milling slugging or formulation. It can affect powder flow properties. It affects the size of high dose capsule product or the homogeneity of a low dose formulation in which there are large differences in drug and excipients densities.

d)Powder flow properties:

The flow properties of powders are critical for an efficient tablet operation. Powders may be free flowing or cohesive (non-free flowing). Flow properties are affected by changes in particle size, density, shape, electrostatic charges, and adsorbed moisture.

e) Compression properties:

The compression properties (elasticity, plasticity, fragment ability and punch filming propensity) for small quantities of a new drug candidate can be established. This property is used in Proper selection of those formulation ingredients were compression properties.

f) Physical description:

It is possible to observe on the bases of size, shape, appearance and determined instrumentally, visually.

3. Solubility analysis:

When the solute dissolves, the substance's inter molecular forces of attraction must be overcome by forces of attraction between solute and solvent molecules. This involves breaking the solute-solute forces and the solvent-solvent forces to achieve the solute-solvent attraction. Methods to improve drug solubility are chemical modification of the drug into salt or ester forms, through selection of a different solubilizing agent, use of co-solvents or other techniques such as micronization or solid dispersion and adjustment of the pH of the solvent in which it is dissolved.

a) Intrinsic Solubility determination:

Steps: I All factors that affect the solubility and drug is to be dissolved.

Steps: II An excess amount of the drug is dispersed in the medium and agitate at constant temperature.

Steps: III Withdraw Samples of the slurry as a function of time.

Steps: IV Clarify Ampoules by filtration or centrifugation.

Steps: V Assay the clear samples for its drug content to establish a plateau concentration and analyze using UV, HPLC, and GC...etc.

b) pKa determination:

Dissociation constant or pKa is usually determined by potentiometric titration. The majority of drugs today are weak organic acids or bases. The concept of pKa is derived from the Henderson-Hasselbalch equation for pKa determination:
For acidic compounds pH= pKa + log (ionized drug/ unionized drug)
For basic compounds pH= Pkw - pKb + log (unionized drug/ionized drug)

c) Partition coefficient:

The oil/water partition coefficient is a measure of a molecule's lipophilic characters that is, its preference for the hydrophilic or lipophilic phase. The partition coefficient should be considered in developing a drug substance into a dosage form. If a solute is added to a mixture of two immiscible liquids, it will distribute between the two phases

and reach equilibrium at a constant temperature. It has a number of applications
1. Used in Solubility determination of both in aqueous and mixed solvents.
2. Partition chromatography can be helpful for column and stationary phase selection (HPLC), choice of plates for TLC and choice of mobile phases (eluents).
3. This information can be effectively used in the extraction of crude drugs.
4. Recovery of antibiotics from fermentation broths and recovery of biotechnology-derived drugs from bacterial cultures.
5. Extraction of drugs from biologic fluids for therapeutic drug monitoring.
6. Absorption of drugs from dosage forms (ointments, supp, TDDS) and study of the distribution of flavoring oil between oil and water phases of emulsions.

d) Dissolution studies:

The speed or rate at which drug substance dissolves in a medium is called dissolution rate. The dissolution rate of the drug in which the surface area is constant during dissolution is described by Noyes Whitney equation.

e) Common ion effect:

The addition of a common ion reduces the solubility of the slightly soluble electrolyte. This salting out (drug precipitation) results from the electrolyte by the hydration of the common ion. Salting in larger anions (hydro tropes) e.g. benzoates, salicylates can open the water molecules allowing an increase in solubility of poorly-water soluble drugs

4. Stability analysis:

a) In toxicology formulations:

These studies are advisable to evaluate samples of toxicology preparations for stability and potential homogeneity problems. Solution and suspension toxicological preparation should be checked for ease of manufacture and stored in flame-sealed ampoules at various temperatures. In chemical stability the suspension should be subjected to an occasional shaking to check dispersibility and drug solubility is analyzed by pH decomposition.

b) Solution stability:

These studies include the effect of pH, Ionic strength, Co-solvent, Light, Temperature.

c) Solid state stability:

It is defined as the capability of a particular formulation in a specific container or closure system to remain within its physical, chemical, microbiological, therapeutic and toxicological specifications. Stability is officially defined as the time lapse during which the drug product retains the same properties and characters that is processed at the time of manufacture. The stability of a product is expressed as the expiry period or technically shelf life. Purpose of stability study to ensure the efficacy, safety, quality of active drug substance and dosage forms, to establish shelf life or expiration period and to support label claims, to gain information about its packaging.

7.2.6 Phytochemical evaluations:

7.2.6.1 Total phenol and flavonoid content:

Test for alkaloids:

To the extracts (0.1 ml), 2 to 3 drops of Dragendroff's reagent were added. An orange red precipitate indicated the presence of alkaloids.

Test for flavonoids:

To the 4mg/ml extract, a piece of magnesium ribbon was added this was followed by concentrated HCl drop. A color change ranging from orange to red indicated flavones while red to crimson indicated flavonoids.

Test for saponins:

To half gram of the extract, five milliliters of distilled water was added to the tubes. A persistent froth that lasts for about 15 min indicated the presence of saponins.

Test for steroids:

To two milliliters of the extract, the residues were dissolved in acetic anhydride and chloroform was then added. This was followed by the addition of concentrated sulfuric acid. A brown ring at the interface of the two liquids and a violet color in the supernatant layer indicated the presence of steroids.

Test for tannins:

To two milliliters of the extract, 2 to 3 drops of 5% ferric chloride was added. A green black or blue coloration indicated the presence of tannins.

Test for glycosides:

To one ml of extract, add ten ml of sulfuric acid. The mixture was heated up to 15min. To that add 10 milliliters Fehling's solution was added. A brick red precipitate indicated presence of glycosides.

Test for terpenoids:

To 0.5 g extract, add 2ml chloroform and 2ml concentrated sulfuric acid. A reddish-brown coloration forms indicated the presence of terpenoids.

Test for phenols:

To the extracts, add few drops of ferric chloride. Formation of bluish black color indicates the presence of phenols.

7.2.7 Qualitative analysis:

It is a process used to determine and identify the physical and chemical properties of an unknown substance.

It is divided into 2 parts:

- ✓ Separation of the different species to avoid interference.
- ✓ Identification step in which chemical reaction are performed with specific reagents.

7.2.8 Quantitative analysis:

It is a process of chemical analysis designed to determine the amounts or proportions of the components of a substance.

7.2.9 Compatibility study: Fourier Transform Infrared Spectroscopy (FTIR):

FTIR spectroscopy can be used to investigate and predict any physicochemical interactions between different components, in a formulation and therefore it can be applied to the selection of suitable chemically compatible excipients. While selecting the vehicle ingredients, we would choose those, which are stable, compatible, cosmetically and therapeutically acceptable.

The aim of the present study was to test, whether there is any interaction between the polymer and the drug and also compatibility between the drug and polymer. 10 mg of the sample and 30 mg of KBr were taken in a mortar and triturated. A small amount of triturated sample was taken into a pellet maker and was compressed at 10 kg/c^2 using a hydraulic press. The pellet was kept on to the sample holder and scanned from 400 cm in Schimadzu FT – IR spectrophotometer.

7.2.10 Formulation of microspheres from the leaves of Musa paradisiaca leaves using Ethyl cellulose carrier (extract: polymers in different ratios) by Solvent Extraction Technique:

Ethyl cellulose microspheres containing Musa paradisiaca leaves extract were prepared in nine different Drug to polymer ratios (1:1, 1:1.5, 1:2, 1:2.5, 1:3, 1:3.5, 1:4, 1:4.5, 1:5) by emulsification and organic solvent evaporation technique. Dissolve specific amount of ethyl cellulose in 20ml of dichloromethane and add slowly 100mg of Musa paradisiaca leaves extract to form uniform solution. Add gradually ethyl cellulose solution containing the drug to beaker containing distilled water and 50ml of 0.5% gelatin solution. The beaker is heated in a water bath at 40°C. The dispersed phase was then added and stirred with using stainless steel mechanical propellar at 2000rpm. Continue mixing (45 min to 60 min) so that all the dichloromethane evaporates. Separate microspheres by filtration using Whatman filter paper and the microspheres thus obtained can be washed four times with 20ml of distilled water and dry in a dessicator. Average particle was determined by using a calibrated stage micrometer and the surface characters were analyzed by scanning electron microscope (SEM).

7.2.11 Evaluation:

❖ **Particle size and shape:**

Optical microscope was used to determine the size of the microspheres. This method involves the calibration of eye piece micrometer for which the stage micrometer is used. In stage micrometer one mm is divided into 100 equal divisions and hence, each division is equal to 10 mm and the particles are measured chosen fixed across the center of the particle. The average diameter was calculated using following formula:

Average diameter = $\sum nd/n \times C.F.$

Where n = number of microspheres,

d = diameter of microspheres,

C.F = calibration factor.

Shape of microspheres was observed by visual observation.

❖ **Percentage yield:**

The dried microspheres were weighed and percentage yield of the prepared microspheres was calculated by using the following formula:

Percentage yield = (Weight of Microspheres – Weight of Polymer + Drug) ×100.

❖ **Drug Entrapment efficiency (DEE%):**

The drug entrapment efficiency of microspheres was determined by taking accurately weighed 100 mg of microspheres in a glass mortar and powdered by a glass pestle and treated with 100 ml of phosphate buffer of Ph 7.4 in a closed volumetric flask and left overnight. Then it was transferred into a 250 ml beaker and stirred by magnetic stirrer using Teflon coated magnetic bead, the temperature was maintained at 37°C±0.5°C. At the end of 1 hour, it was centrifuged and supernatant was filtered, the filtrate was analyzed spectrophotometrically at 284 nm. Dilution was done whenever required using phosphate buffer Ph 7.4. Corresponding drug concentrations in samples was calculated from calibration plot. Entrapment efficiency of the microspheres was calculated using the formula:

DEE% = Practical drug loading / Theoretical drug loading × 100.

❖ **Scanning electron microscope study:**

The microspheres were observed under a scanning electron microscope. The instrument used for the study was Hitachi S- 450 scanning electron microscope. The microspheres were mounted directly on to the SEM sample stub, using double sided sticking tape, and coated with gold film (thickness 200 nm) under reduced pressure (0.001 torr).

❖ **FTIR spectra analysis:**

FTIR spectroscopy can be used to investigate and predict any physicochemical interactions between different components, in a formulation and therefore it can be applied to the selection of suitable chemically compatible excipients. While selecting the vehicle ingredients, we could choose those, which are stable, compatible, cosmetically and therapeutically acceptable.

The aim of the present study was to test, whether there is any interaction between the polymer and the drug and also compatibility between the drug and polymer.

10 mg of the sample and 30 mg of KBr were taken in a mortar and triturated. A small amount of triturated sample was taken into a pellet maker and was compressed at

10 kg/c^2 using a hydraulic press. The pellet was kept on to the sample holder and scanned from 4000cm to 400cm in Schimadzu FT-IR spectrophotometer.

MICROMERITICS:

Microparticles are characterized by their micromeritic properties like bulk density, tapped density, angle of repose and compressibility index.

❖ **Bulk density:**

An accurately weighed sample of microspheres was carefully introduced into a 10 ml graduated cylinder with the aid of funnel. Typically, the initial volume was noted.

Carefully level the microspheres without copacting, if necessary, and read the unsettled apparent volume VO, to the nearest graduated unit. Calculate the bulk density in g/cm^3 by the formula.

$D_f = M/V_O$

Where D_f= bulk density,

M = weight of samples in grams,

VO = volume of sample in cm^3.

- **Tapped density:**

A required quantity of microspheres from each formula was introduced into a measuring cylinder. After the initial volume was observed, the cylinder was allowed to fall under its own weight onto a hard surface from the height of 2.5 cm at 2sec interval. The tapping was continued until no further change in volume was noted. Tapped density were calculated using the following formula:

Tapped density = W/V_f

Where W = weight of the powder,

V_o = initial volume

V_f = final volume.

- **Swelling index:**

The accurately weighed dried microspheres were placed in USP dissolution apparatus II containing 900 ml, phosphate buffer (pH 6.8) maintained at 37± 2°C and allowed to swell up to constant weight. The microspheres were removed, blotted with filter paper, and changes in weight were measured. The experiments were carried out in triplicate. The degree of swelling (Swelling index) was then calculated from the formula:

Swelling index = $(W_g - W_o) \times 100 / W_o$

Where, W_O = initial weight of microspheres,

W_g = weight of microspheres at equilibrium swelling in the medium.

FLOW PROPERTIES:

The flow characterstics are measured by angle of repose and compressibility index. Improper flow of powder due to frictional forces is quantified by angle of repose.

❖ **Angle of repose:**

Angle of repose was determined by using funnel method, the accurately weighed spheres were taken in funnel. The height of funnel was adjusted in such a way that the tip of funnel just touches the apex of heap of blends. The blends were allowed to flow through funnel freely on to surface. The diameter of powder cone was measured, angle of repose was calculated by using following equation:

$$\text{Tan } \Theta = h/r$$

Where, h = height of pile,

r = radius of base pile,

Θ = angle of repose

Table 3: Angle of Repose and its properties

Angle of repose	Properties
< 25	Excellent flow
25 – 30	Good flow
30 – 40	Passable
>40	Very poor flow

❖ **Compressibility index %:**

It is one of method for determining flow properties and also called as Carr's index of compressibility. It is indirectly related to the relative flow rate, cohesiveness and particle size. It is simple, fast and popular method of predicting powder flow characterstics.

$$C_I = 100\,(V_O - V_f) / V_O$$

Table 4: % Compressibility index and its properties

% Comp. Index	Properties
5 – 12	Free flowing
12 – 16	Good
18 – 21	Fair

23 - 35	Poor
33 - 38	Very poor
>40	Extremely poor

7.2.12 Study of the invitro release pattern of drug from ethyl cellulose microspheres containing Musa paradisiaca leaves extract:

The drug release study was performed using USP type XXIII dissolution test apparatus, paddle model and at 100rpm using 900ml of phosphate buffer saline 7.4 pH as a dissolution medium. The medium temperature was maintained at 37±0.5°C. Periodically 1ml of samples were withdrawn and diluted to 10ml by using phosphate buffer pH 7.4. After each withdrawal the same quantity of the fresh medium was replaced immediately. Then the samples were assayed spectrophotometrically, Schimadzu Pharmaspec 1700 UV spectrophotometer at 496nm using medium as blank.

7.2.13 Stability studies of ethyl cellulose microspheres containing Musa paradisiaca leaves extract:

All the formulations were studied for stability profile for 1 month at different environmental conditions such as 4°C, 25°C and 45°C. The microspheres were placed in screw capped glass containers and stored at ambient temperatures by keeping the microspheres in refrigerator to produce 4°C environment, 45°Cenvironment was produced by keeping the microspheres in hot air oven. From the above samples every week up to one-month period suitable representative samples were taken and it is analyzed for drug content. Change in average drug content was noted.

8.RESULTS AND DISCUSSION

The sustained release microspheres of Musa paradisiaca were prepared by using ethyl cellulose and evaluated with an aim to prevent side effects and increase bioavailability. It also leads to reduction in frequency of dosing which in turn improves patient compliance and reduce fluctuation in drug levels. Prepared Musa paradisiaca microspheres were subjected to various evaluation parameters such as FTIR characterization, size determination by microscopic method, shape and surface determination by digital photography, micromeritics properties like bulk density, tapped density, flow property by angle of repose, encapsulation efficiency determination and in-vitro dissolution studies.

8.1 SELECTION OF WAVELENGTH:

The extract solution (5, 10, 15, 20, 25µg/mL) in distilled water was taken in a standard cuvette and scanned in the range of 200 – 450 nm in UV spectrophotometer. It exhibits maxima at 450 nm. The absorption peak obtained is

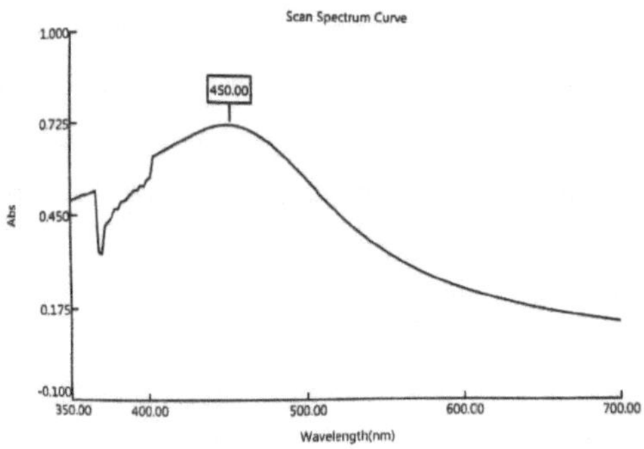

Fig 12: UV spectra of Musa paradisiaca extract

8.2 PHYTOCHEMICAL STUDIES:

Table 5: Phytochemical constituents

S. No.	Chemical constituents	Ethanolic Extract
1.	Alkaloids	+
2.	Saponins	+
3.	Tannins	+
4.	Flavonoids	+
5.	Terpenoids	+
6.	Steroids	+
7.	Phenol	+
8.	Phlobatannins	+
9.	Cardiac glycosides	+

The phytochemical studies revealed the presence of alkaloids, flavonoids, phenolic compounds, glycosides and steroids.

8.3 COMPATIBILITY STUDIES BY FTIR:

8.3.1 FTIR Studies:

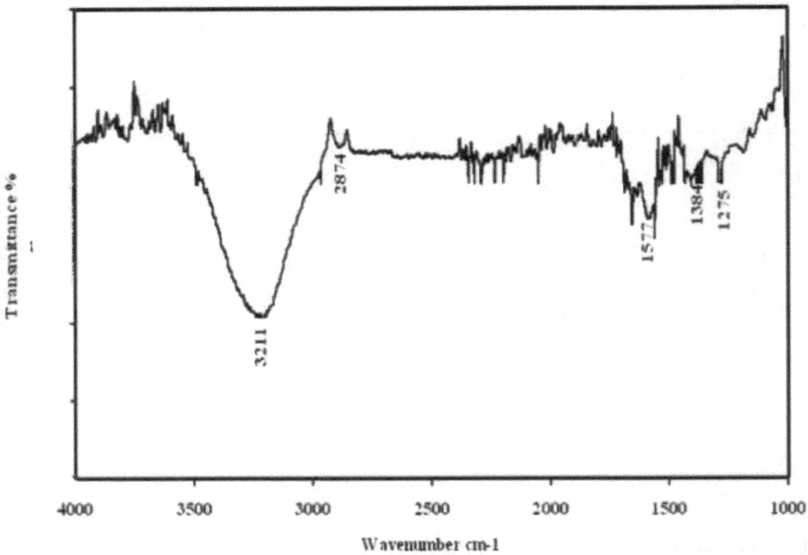

Fig 13: FTIR Spectra of Musa paradisiaca extract

Table 6: FTIR Interpretation of Musa paradisiaca extract

Wave number (cm^{-1})	Functional groups
3211.65	0-H stretching
2874.14	C-H stretching
1384.93	C-H bending
1275.54	C-O stretching

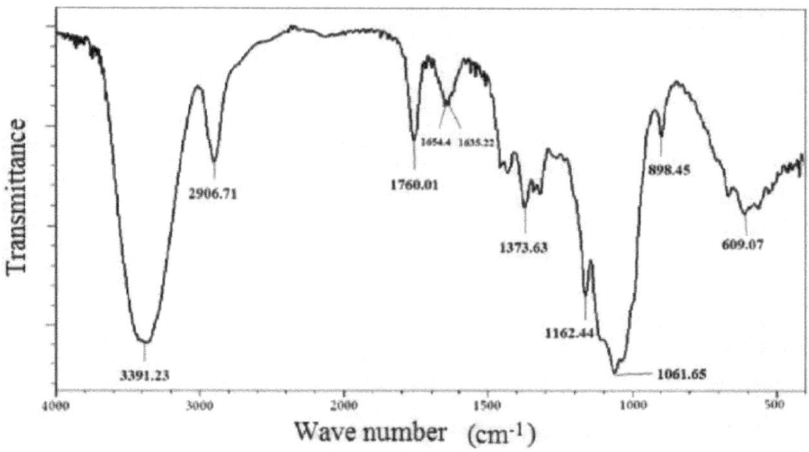

Fig 14: FTIR Spectra of Ethyl Cellulose

Table 7: FTIR Interpretation of Ethyl Cellulose

Wave number (cm^{-1})	Functional groups
3391.23	- OH stretching
2906.71	C-H bending
1760.01	C=C stretching
1061.65	C-C Stretching
898.45	C-H bending
609.07	C-X stretching

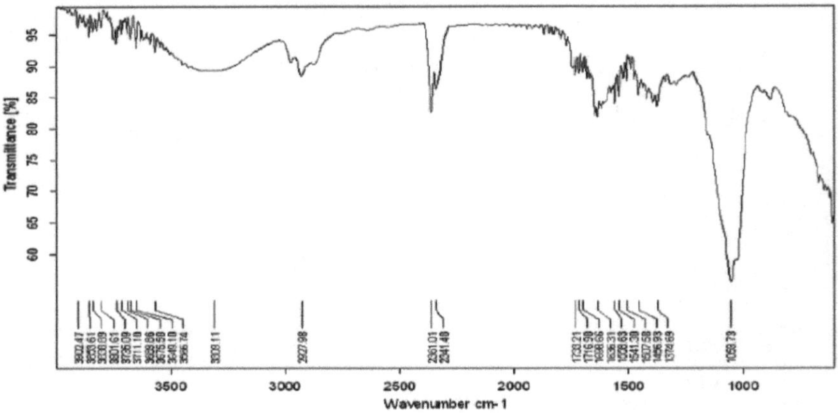

Fig 15: FTIR Spectra of physical mixture of Musa paradisiaca extract using Ethyl Cellulose

Table 8: FTIR Interpretation of physical mixture of Musa paradisiaca using Ethyl Cellulose

Wave number (cm^{-1})	Functional groups
3302.47	0-H stretching
3303.61	0-H stretching
3000.89	C-H stretching
1507.58	$N0_2$ stretching
1456.93	C-H bending
1374.69	C-O stretching
1063.78	O-H bending

The drug was identified and confirmed by an IR spectrum. Fig.12 shows the IR spectrum of Musa paradisiaca extract. Fig. 13 shows the IR spectrum of Ethyl Cellulose. Fig. 14 shows the IR spectrum of the physical mixture of Musa paradisiaca extract using Ethyl Cellulose. From the spectrum, it was concluded the incorporation pf the drug in to the polymer didn't change the characterstics of the drug.

8.4 STANDARD CURVE OF SYNTHETIC DRUG:

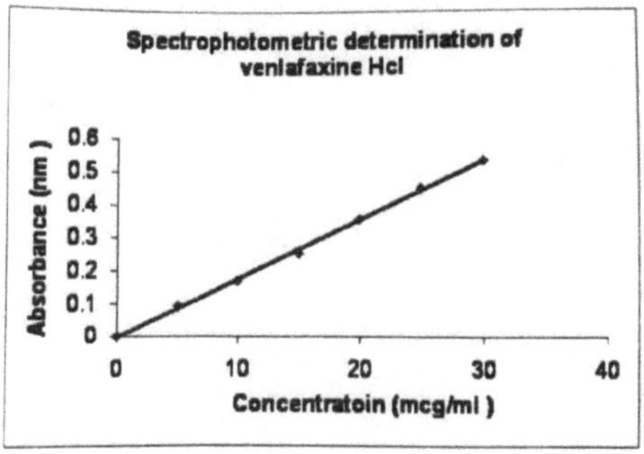

Fig 16: Standard Curve of Venlafaxine Hydrochloride

Table no. 9 and fig no.14 shows the standard curve of Venlafaxine Hydrochloride. The method was validated for linearity, accuracy and precision. The method obeyed Beer's law in the concentration range of 5- 30 μg/ ml.

Table 9: Standard Curve of Venlafaxine Hydrochloride

S. NO	Concentration (μg/ ml)	Absorbance (496nm)
1	0	0
2	5	0.089
3	10	0.15
4	15	0.259
5	20	0.361
6	25	0.449
7	30	0.556

8.5 EVALUATION:

8.5.1 Particle Size and Shape:

8.5.2 Percentage Yield and Drug Entrapment Efficiency:

It is essential to know the quantity of the drug entrapped in the microspheres before going to study the behaviors of this drug in physical or biological system. The percentage of entrapment was determined for all the batches and it was shown in table 10. The encapsulation efficiency was in the range of 69.8 – 76.1% with various batches. Drug content of the microspheres was found to be nearly same in all nine batches.

Table 10: Theoretical Drug Content, Estimated Drug Content and Drug

Entrapment Efficiency of Microspheres of Musa paradisiaca

S.No	Formulation code	Theoretical Drug Content In (mg)	Estimated Drug Content In (mg)	Entrapment Efficiency %
1	FE1	42.0	29.3	69.8
2	FE2	52.4	36.9	70.4
3	FE3	65.7	46.9	71.3
4	FE4	89.5	64.5	72.1
5	FE5	95.6	69.3	72.4
6	FE6	95.9	70.2	73.2
7	FE7	94.8	70.7	74.6
8	FE8	96.9	72.9	75.2
9	FE9	99.3	75.6	76.1

Table 11: Percentage Yield of Microspheres

S. No	Formulation code	Percentage Yield
1	FE1	91.0
2	FE2	92.8
3	FE3	93.4
4	FE4	94.0
5	FE5	94.6
6	FE6	96.6
7	FE7	95.8
8	FE8	97.0
9	FE9	98.3

8.5.3 Scanning Electron Microscope Study:

The scanning electron microscopy of the microspheres was shown in below figure. Most of the microspheres were spherical in shape and size ranges from 10 - 100μm. Only some spheres were larger in size. The size distribution of the microspheres was found to be normal in all the batches.

MICROMERITICS:

Micromeritics investigations such as bulk density, tapped density, angle of repose and % compressibility index were carried out on Musa paradisiaca microspheres in order to standardize the product and to optimize the pilot production of dosage forms. Above mentioned properties are studied to determine compressibility and flow properties, the results are tabulated as in Table 13. The values for bulk density and tapped density are shown in table 12. The angle of repose for microsphere was found to be 21°12', 22°21', 23°43', 24°54', 25°41', 26°42', 27°25', 29°46' and 30°27' for the formulation FE1, FE2, FE3, FE4, FE5, FE6, FE7, FE8 and FE9. The result showed the angle of repose is less than 35° and compressibility index also lie between 9.17 and 13.30, which indicate good flow properties. The flowability of microspheres were found to bE according to Carr's index of compressibility. The results were confirmed by relationship between angle of repose (Θ) and Carr's index. The above micromeritic studies show that the prepared microspheres were spherical, non – aggregated and uniform in size and also have compressibility and flowability properties.

8.5.4 and 8.5.5 Bulk Density and Tapped Density:

Table 12: Bulk density and tapped density of microspheres of Musa paradisiaca

S. No	Formulation code	Bulk Density	Tapped Density
1	FE1	0.74 ± 0.010	**0.89 ± 0.024**
2	FE2	0.76 ± 0.010	**0.89 ± 0.038**
3	FE3	0.78 ± 0.033	**0.90 ± 0.039**
4	FE4	0.79 ± o.024	**0.91 ± 0.025**
5	FE5	0.80 ± 0.020	**0.91 ± 0.051**
6	FE6	0.87 ± 0.033	**0.96 ± 0.039**
7	FE7	0.91 ± 0.024	**1.09 ± 0.025**
8	FE8	0.93 ± 0.045	**1.10 ± 0.022**
9	FE9	0.97 ± 0.015	**1.16 ± 0.038**

*Average of Three Determinations

± Standard Deviation

8.5.6 and 8.5.7 Angle of Repose and % Compressibility Index:

Table 13: Angle of Repose and % Compressibility index of microspheres of Musa paradisiaca

S. No	Formulation code	Angle of Repose	% Compressibility index
1	FE1	21° 12'	13.30
2	FE2	22° 21'	12.14
3	FE3	23° 43'	9.24
4	FE4	24° 54'	13.30
5	FE5	25° 41'	9.76
6	FE6	26° 42'	12.29
7	FE7	27° 25'	13.14
8	FE8	29° 46'	13.90
9	FE9	30° 27'	9.17

8.6 STUDY OF THE INVITRO RELEASE PATTERN OF DRUG FROM ETHYL CELLULOSE MICROSPHERES CONTAINING MUSA PARADISIACA LEAF EXTRACT:

The in vitro studies of Musa paradisiaca ethyl cellulose microspheres were determined by Invitro dissolution method, containing 900ml of dissolution medium as phosphate buffer pH 7.4. The microsphere formulation of Musa paradisiaca using ethyl cellulose retards the release of Musa paradisiaca from the microsphere and produces the sustained action. The microspheres prepared with the core: coat ratio of 1:1 release 90.46% of Musa paradisiaca atb24 hours and 1:1.5, 1:2, 1:2.5, 1:3, 1:3.5,1:4, 1:4.5 and 1:5 ethyl cellulose microsphere releases the drug Musa paradisiaca at 24hrs respectively. The increase in concentration of ethyl cellulose causes the decreasing rate of drug release. The release was depended on the core: coat ratio and size of the microspheres. The invitro release profile of the microspheres are tabulated in table 14 – 22 and fig 16 – 24.

Table 14: Invitro release profile of microspheres (FE1) of Musa paradisiaca

Time (Hrs)	Cumulative % drug release
0	0.000
3	21.126
6	37.762
9	47.623
12	50.978
15	63.211
18	78.201
21	86.710
24	90.326

Fig 16: Invitro release profile of microspheres (FE1) of Musa paradisiaca

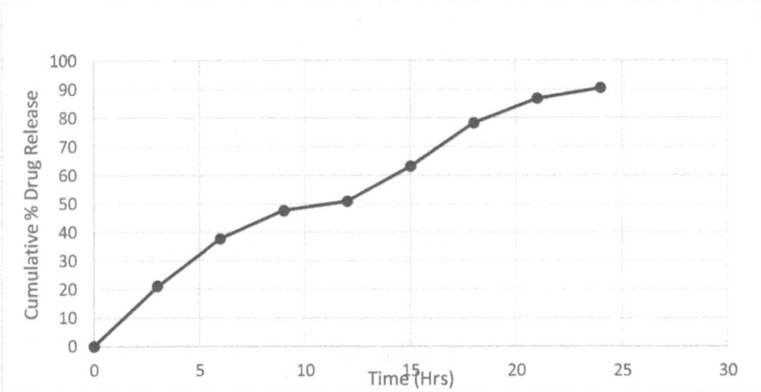

Table 15: Invitro release profile of microspheres (FE2) of Musa paradisiaca

Time (Hrs)	Cumulative % drug release
0	0.000
3	20.120
6	36.293
9	45.967
12	49.627
15	59.091
18	77.665
21	83.002
24	88.326

Fig 17: Invitro release profile of microspheres (FE2) of Musa paradisiaca

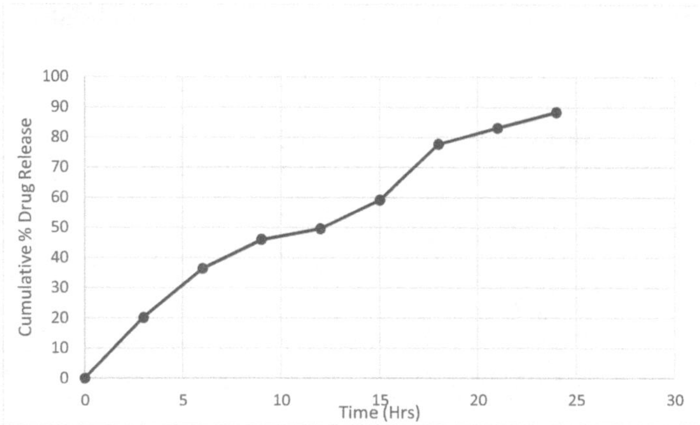

Table 16: Invitro release profile of microspheres (FE3) of Musa paradisiaca

Time (Hrs)	**Cumulative % drug release**
0	0.000
3	19.711
6	35.564
9	41.272
12	47.119
15	58.057
18	69.160
21	80.111
24	86.831

Fig 18: Invitro release profile of microspheres (FE3) of Musa paradisiaca

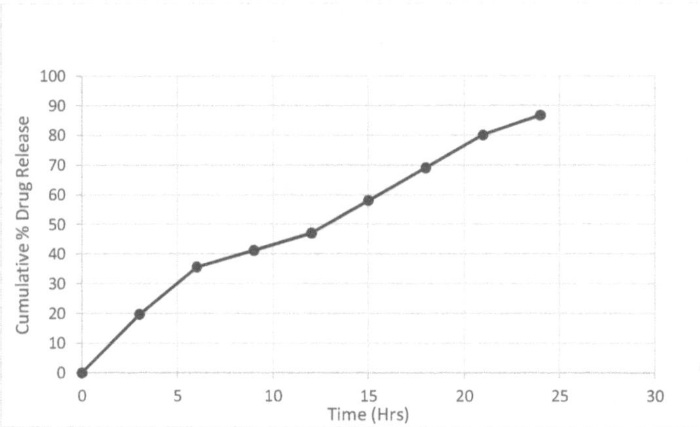

Table 17: Invitro release profile of microspheres (FE4) of Musa paradisiaca

Time (Hrs)	Cumulative % drug release
0	0.000
3	18.048
6	32.357
9	40.828
12	45.105
15	56.268
18	70.877
21	80.639
24	85.403

Fig 19: Invitro release profile of microspheres (FE4) of Musa paradisiaca

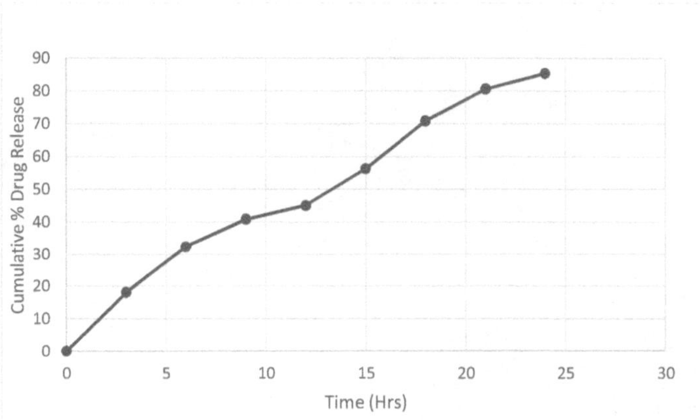

Table 18: In vitro release profile of microspheres (FE5) of Musa paradisiaca

Time (Hrs)	Cumulative % drug release
0	0.000
3	18.137
6	31.125
9	40.010
12	42.489
15	55.794
18	68.631
21	79.465
24	84.377

Fig 20: In vitro release profile of microspheres (FE5) of Musa paradisiaca

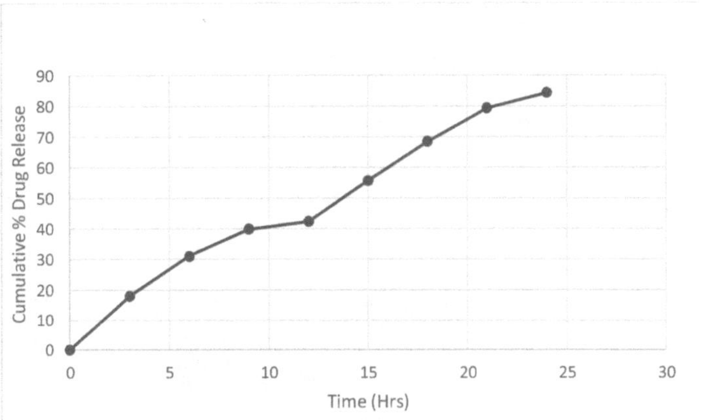

Table 19: Invitro release profile of microspheres (FE6) of Musa paradisiaca

Time (Hrs)	Cumulative % drug release
0	0.000
3	14.508
6	30.800
9	36.687
12	42.567
15	52.982
18	66.914
21	76.649
24	80.569

Fig 21: Invitro release profile of microspheres (FE6) of Musa paradisiaca

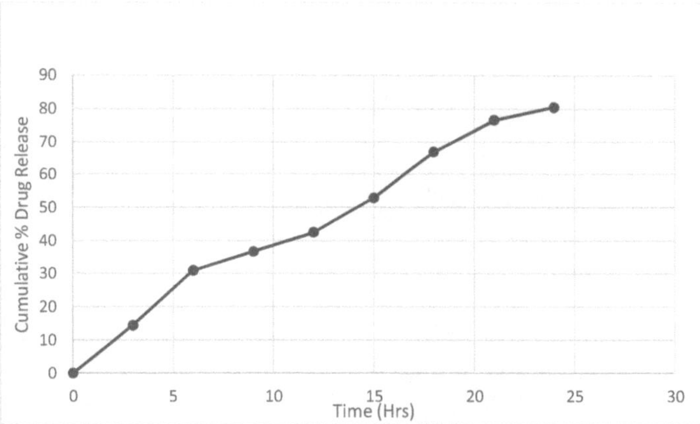

Table 20: Invitro release profile of microspheres (FE7) of Musa paradisiaca

Time (Hrs)	Cumulative 5 drug release
0	0.000
3	20.465
6	35.527
9	43.274
12	49.412
15	60.211
18	70.446
21	81.273

24	88.564

Fig 22: Invitro release profile of microspheres (FE7) of Musa paradisiaca

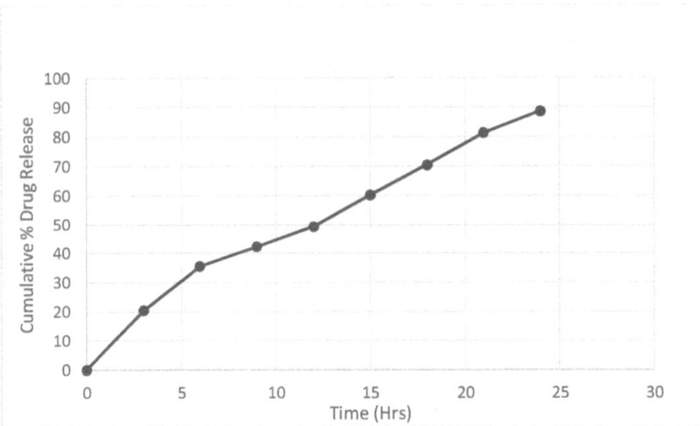

Table 21: Invitro release profile of microspheres (FE8) of Musa paradisiaca

Time (Hrs)	Cumulative % drug release
0	0.000
3	21.424
6	38.280
9	48.565
12	50.227
15	61.726
18	78.161

21	85.765
24	88.665

Fig 23: Invitro release profile of microspheres (FE8) of Musa paradisiaca

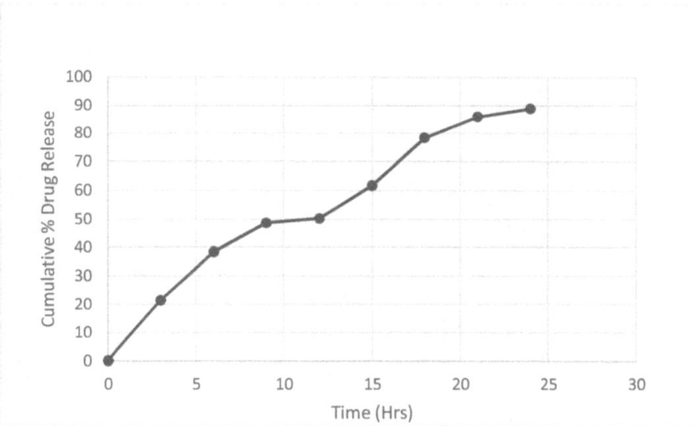

Table 22: Invitro release profile of microspheres (FE9) of Musa paradisiaca

Time (Hrs)	Cumulative % drug release
0	0.000
3	21.424
6	38.280
9	47.565
12	50.227
15	60.726

18	78.161
21	85.765
24	89.665

Fig 24: Invitro release profile of microspheres (FE9) of Musa paradisiaca

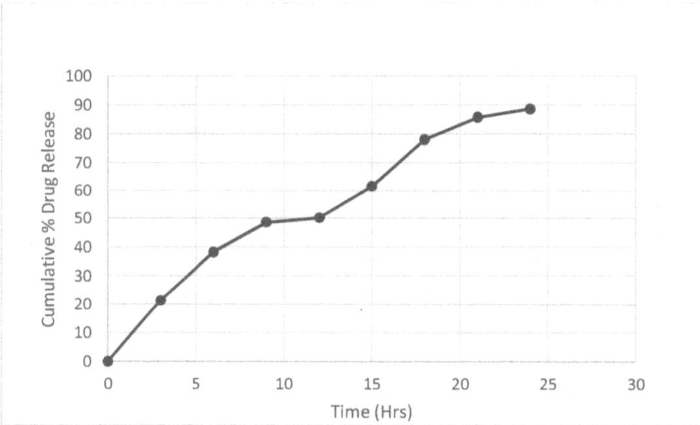

Fig 25: Invitro release profile of microspheres of Musa paradisiaca (FE1- FE9)

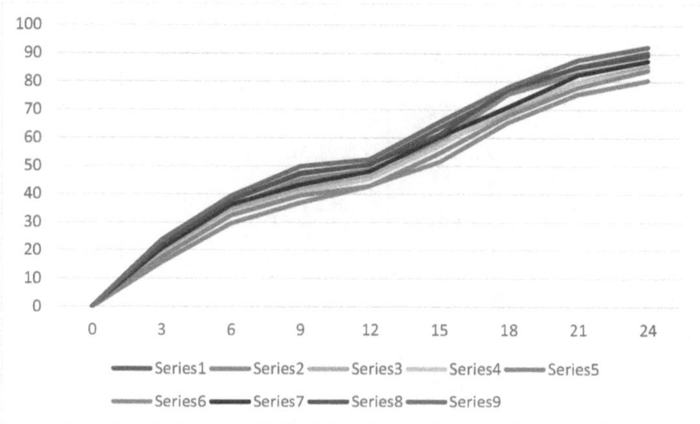

INVITRO KINETIC PROFILE FOR FORMULATION (FE 9):

FORMULATION CODE	TIME (IN Hrs)	S.Q.R.T OF TIME	Log TIME	CUMULATIVE % DRUG RELEASE	Log Cumulative % DRUG RELEASE
	0	0			
	3	1.732	0.477		
	6	2.449	0.788		
	9	3	0.954		

FE 9	12	3.464	1.079		
	15	3.872	1.176		
	18	4.242	1.255		
	21	4.582	1.322		
	24	4.898	1.380		

8.7 STABILITY STUDIES OF ETHYL CELLULOSE MICROSPHERES CONTAINING MUSA PARADISIACA EXTRACT:

Physical stability and effect on the drug release were studied in the microspheres, all microsphere formulations were kept in the small air tight glass containers and stored at different temperatures at 4°C in a refrigerator, 25°C and 45°C in the oven, effect on their release characterstics was studied every week up to one moth by using dissolution method.

Table no.23 shows the stability of microsphere formulation at various temperatures like 4°C, 25°C, 45°C, there was no significant change in the release pattern when it was stored at 4°C, 25°C and slightly affected in 45°C.

Table 23: The stability of Microsphere formulation at various temperatures

Fc	Refrigeration Temp. (4^0 C)				Room Temp (25°C)				High Temp (45°C)			
	DAYS				DAYS				DAYS			
	7	14	21	28	7	14	21	28	7	14	21	28
FE1	100	98.1	96.4	96.3	96.4	95.3	92	90.8	85	82.2	81.4	80
FE2	100	98.2	96.5	96.4	96.6	95.5	93.5	91.3	85.5	82.5	81.7	80.6
FE3	100	98.3	96.9	96.5	97	95.9	93.7	91.5	85.7	82.9	82.9	82.3
FE4	100	98.4	97.3	96.7	97.3	96.1	94	91.7	85.9	83.3	83.8	82.9
FE5	100	98.5	97.4	96.9	97.6	96.3	94.3	92	86	83.9	84.1	83.2
FE6	100	98.6	97.7	97	97.8	96.5	94.4	92.5	86.4	84.1	84.6	83.7
FE7	100	99.3	97.9	97.3	98.5	97.3	95.6	93.8	86.8	84.2	83.8	82.9
FE8	100	99.6	98.6	98.3	98.7	96	95.3	94.4	87.3	85	84.1	83
FE9	100	99.9	98.8	98.4	100	99.5	98.3	96.6	88.7	86.5	84.4	83.5

9. SUMMARY AND CONCLUSION

Formulation FE9 was found to be the optimized formulation out of nine formulations potentially due to high concentration of the polymer Ethyl Cellulose. The drug release of FE9 in 24 hours is found to be 89.665% which was the highest among the formulations carried out.

During the last two decades much attention has been given to the design of controlled drug delivery system that increase the effectiveness of the existing drugs, use of this approach has the potential not only to improve the therapeutic effectiveness of the drug but also to follow a reduction in the total drug needed and minimizing toxic side effects. Microspheres are one of the devices that have been used for the delivery of drugs to affected area. Microspheres are relatively non- toxic and non—immunogenic preparations made to reduce the gap between the sustained release preparations and controlled release preparations. In the present study, an attempt was made to develop a new sustained drug delivery for Musa paradisiaca microspheres by using Ethyl Cellulose to improve patient compliance and safety.

In this present work, the first chapter deals with the introduction of sustained release technology, microspheres, diabetes and anti- diabetic. The second chapter deals with literature review. The third chapter deals with aim and objective. The fourth chapter contains plan of work. The fifth and sixth chapter deals with details about the drug Musa paradisiaca and polymer Ethyl Cellulose. The seventh chapter deals with entire methodology of the work. The microspheres were prepared by emulsification and organic solvent evaporation method and characterized by using scanning electron microscope, sustained release formulation of Musa paradisiaca in the form of microspheres was developed to a satisfactory level in term of drug release, content uniformity and micromeritics properties. The compatibility studies were done by FTIR spectroscopy. It implies that there was no interaction between drug and polymers and they are compatible with each other. The micromeritics data showed that there was not much significant difference in term of angle of repose, bulk density, size distribution by microscopic method showed not much significant difference in formulations but increasing the concentration of polymer increased the size range.

The in vitro release profile of microspheres in phosphate buffer pH at 37°C confirmed the sustained release of microspheres, the increasing concentration of polymer is decreased in the release rate. In conclusion, it is possible to prepare microspheres containing Musa paradisiaca by emulsification and organic solvent evaporation method, to prolonged activity with increased stability without losing its therapeutic activity. Further work is required for in vivo studies, estimate the amount of drug present in the various organs with disposition kinetics and establish appropriate dosage regimens to gauge the significant changes in the metabolism of drug before studies in the clinic.

10. REFERENCES

1. Ramteke K.H, Jadhav V.B, Dhole S.N. Microspheres: as carriers used for novel drug delivery system IOSR Journal of Pharmacy (IOSRPHR) ISSN: 2250-3013, Vol. 2, Issue 4 (July 2012), PP 44-48.
2. M. Alagu sundaram, Madhu Sudana Chetty et al. Microsphere as A Novel Drug Delivery System A Review. International Journal of Chem Tech Research. 2009;1(3):526-534.
3. B. Sree Giri Prasad, V. R. M Gupta, N. Devana, K. Jayasurya, Microspheres as Drug Delivery System – A Review Journal of Global Trends in Pharmaceutical Sciences.
4. S. Davis, L. Ilum, microspheres as a drug carrier in "drug carrier system", F.H. Roerdnik and A.M.Kron (Eds), John Wiley and sons ltd 1989, page no.1 5.
5. Chowdary KPR, Yaraguntla SR. Mucoadhesive microsphere for controlled drug delivery. Biol. Pharm. Bull. 2004;1717.
6. 6. Shanthi NC, Gupta R, Mahato KA, Traditional and Emerging Applications of Microspheres: A Review, International Journal of Pharm. Tech Research. 2010; 2(1):675- 691.
7. Najmudin M., Ahmed A., Shelar S, Patel V, Khan T. Floating Microspheres of Ketoprofen: Formulation and Evaluation, International Journal of Pharmacy and Pharmaceutical sciences. 2010; 2(2):83-87.
8. Yadav AV, Mote HH. Development of Biodegradable Starch Microspheres for Intranasal Delivery, Indian Journal of pharmaceutical Sciences. 2008; 70 (2):170-74.
9. Dandagi MP, Masthiolimath SV, Gadad PA, Iliger R.S. Mucoadhesive Microspheres of Propanalol Hcl for Nasal Delivery, Indian Journal of pharmaceutical Sciences. 2007;69 (3): 402.
10. Pradesh TS, Sunny M., Varma KH, Ramesh P. Preparation of micro structured hydroxyapatite microspheres using oil in water emulsion, Bull Matter. Sci. 2005; 28(5): 383- 90.
11. Venkatesh H. (1989) "A buccal delivery system of Salbutamol Sulphate" M. Pharm; Budrinarayan N. (1991) "Utilization and Evaluation of plant products in pharmaceutical formulations". M. Pharm.
12. Save T, Venkatachalam P. "Bio-adhesive tablets of Nifedipine: Standardization of a novel Bucco adhesive erodible carrier". Drug Delivery. Ind. pharm. 1994;20(19): 3005-14.

13. Lopez CR, Portero A, Vila-Jato JC, Alonso MJ. "Design and Evaluation of Chitosan/Ethyl cellulose mucoadhesive bi-layered devices for buccal drug delivery". J. control. Rel. 1998;55: 143-52.
14. Alagusundaram M, Chetty MSC, Uma shankari K, Badrinath AV, Lavanya C, Ramkanth S. Microspheres as a Novel Drug Delivery System- A Review. Int. J. of Chem. Tech Res. 2009;1: 526-34.
15. Rathone MJ. "Human buccal absorption. A method for Estimating the transfer kinetics of drugs across the human buccal membrane". Int. J. pharm. 1991;69: 103.
16. Rathone MJ. (1991a) "Human buccal absorption I.A method for Estimating the transfer kinetics of drugs across the human buccal membrane". Int. J. pharm. (1991a) 69:103.
17. Nachts S and Martin K. In: The microsponges, novel topical programmable delivery formulation, Marcel Dekker Inc. New York. 1990; 299.
18. Hafeli U. Physics and Chemistry Basic of Biotechnology: Focus on biotechnology. Review: Radioactive Microspheres for Medical Application, 7:213-248.
19. Adewoye, E.O., V.O. Taiwo and Olayioye, F.A. 2010. Anti-oxidant and anti-hyperglycemic activities of Musa sapientum root extracts in alloxan induced diabetic rats. J Med Chem. 28;53(20):7365-76.
20. Dhanabal, S.P., M. Suresh kumar, M. Ramanathan and Suresh, B. 2010. Hypoglycemic effect of ethanolic extract of Musa sapientum on alloxan induced diabetes mellitus in rats and its relation with antioxidant potential. J Nutr. 140(8):1462-8.
21. Entaz Bahar, Joushan Ara, Mofasser Hossain and Obayed Raihan. 2013. Antioxidant (In-Vitro) Effect of Methanol& Petroleum Ether Extracts of the Aerva lanata. The pharma innovation. IC Journal No: 7725, Vol. 2.
22. Jamuna, J., Mysore Shobha, Kari Sambaiah and Paramahans Salimath. 2011. Beneficial effects of banana (Musa sp. var. elakki bale) flower and pseudo-stem on hyperglycemia and advanced glycation end-products (AGEs) in streptozotocin-induced diabetic rats. J Physio Bio-chem. 67(3):415-25.
23. Lewis, D.A., W.N. Fields and Shaw, G.P. 1999. A natural flavonoid present in unripe plantain banana pulp (Musa sapientum L. var. paradisiaca) protects the gastric mucosa from aspirin induced erosions. J Ethnopharmacol. 65(3):283-8.
24. Makkar, H.P.S., M. Bluemmel, N.K. Borowy and Becker, K. 1993. Gravimetric determination of tannins and their correlations with chemical and protein precipitation methods. J. Sci. Food Agric. 61: 161 165.

25. Mukhopadhyay, S., D. L. Luthria and Robbins R. 2006. Optimization of Extraction Process for Phenolic Acids from Black Cohosh (Cimicifuga racemosa) by Pressurized Liquid Extraction. J. Sci. Food Agric. 86: 156 162.
26. Nicholson, R.L. and Hammer schmidt, R. 1992. Phenolic Compounds and Their Role in Disease Resistance. Annual Review of Phytopathology. Vol. 30: 369-389.
27. Raji, R. and Raveendran, K. 2013. Antifungal activity of selected plant extracts against phytopathogenic fungi Aspergillus niger. Asian Journal of Plant Science and Research. 3(1):13- 15.
28. Suhad Humadi and Viorica Istudor. 2009. Lythrum salicaria (Purple loosestrife). Medicinal use, extraction and identification of its total phenolic compounds. Farmacia. Vol. 57, 192- 200. 62.Thakorlal, J., C.O. Perera, B. Smith, L. Englberger and Lorens, A. 2010. Resistant starch in Micronesian banana cultivars offers health benefits. Pac Health Dialog. 16(1):49-59.
29. Venkatesan K, Manavalan R, Valliapan K. 2009. Microencapsulation: a vital technique in novel drug delivery system. J Pharm Sci Res. 1(4): 26-35.
30. Ghulam M, Mahmood A, Naveed A, Fatima R.2009. Comparative study of various microencapsulation techniques. Effect of polymer viscosity on microcapsule characteristics, Pak. J. Sci. 22 (3):291-300.
31. Mathew T, Devi S, Prasanth V, Vinod B. 2010. Suitability of factorial design in determining the processing factors affecting entrapment efficiency of albumin microspheres. J Pharm Res. 3(5):1172- 1177.
32. CA 2579533, Andrew Lennard Lewis Peter William Stratford Maria Victoria Gonzalez-
Fajardo Yiqing Tang, Publication: 06-09-05.
33. Kavita K, Raje V, et al. 2010. Albumin Microspheres: A Unique system as drug delivery carriers for non- steroidal anti-inflammatory drugs. 5(2):12.
34. Khar R.K, Vyas, S.P. 2002. Targeted and Controlled Drug Delivery- Novel Carrier Systems., 1st edition, CBS Publications and Distributors, New Delhi ;417- 418.
35. Li S.P, Kowalski C.R, Feld K.M, Grim W.M. 1988. Recent Advances in Microencapsulation Technology and Equipment, Drug Dev Ind Pharm. 14: 353-376.
36. Shanthi N.C, Gupta R, Mahato K.A. 2010 Traditional and Emerging Applications of Microspheres: A Review, International Journal of Pharm Tech Research. 2(1):675-681. =90. Floating Microspheres of Ketoprofen: Formulation and Evaluation, International Journal of Pharmacy and Pharmaceutical sciences. 2(2):83-87.

37. http://www.springerlink.com /content/r883r91q17576vx6/ DOI: 10.1007/0-306-46891-3_9, Hafeli U, 2002, Physics and Chemistry Basic of Biotechnology. Focus on biotechnology. Review. Radioactive Microspheres for Medical Application, 7:213-248.
38. Yadav AV, Mote HH. 2008. Development of Biodegradable Starch Microspheres for Intranasal Delivery, Indian Journal of pharmaceutical Sciences. 70 (2):170-174.
39. Saralidze K, Leo H, Koole, Menno L, Knetsch W. 2010. Polymeric Microspheres for Medical Applications, Materials. 3:3357- 3564.
40. Trivedi P, Verma L, Garud N. 2008.Preparation and Characterization of Aceclofenac Microspheres, Asian Journal of pharmaceutics. 2(2): 110-115.
41. Alagusundaram M, Madhu C, Uma shankari K, Attuluri B, Lavanya C, Ramkanth S. Microspheres: As novel drug delivery system. International Journal of Chem Tech Research. 2009; 1(3): 526-534.
42. Kannan.K., Karar.K.P., Manavalan.R., Formulation and Evaluation of Sustained Release Microspheres of Acetazolamide by Solvent Evaporation Technique, J. Pharm. Sci& Res. 2009; 1 (1):36-39.
43. Shaji J., Poddar A., Iyer S., Brain-Targeted Nasal Clonazepam Microspheres, Indian Journal of pharmaceutical Sciences. 2009; 71(6): 715–719.
44. Chowdary K.P.R., Suri B.J., Permeability of Ethylene Vinyl Acetate Copolymer Microcapsules: Effect of Solvents, Indian Journal of pharmaceutical Sciences. 2003; 65(1):62-66.
45. Soni L.M., Kumar M., Namdeo P.K., Sodium alginate Microspheres for extending drug release: formulation and in vitro evaluation, International Journal of Drug Delivery. 2010; 2(1):64-68.
46. Surini S., Anggriani V., Anwar E., Study of Mucoadhesive Microspheres Based on Pre-gelatinized Cassava Starch Succinate as a New Carrier for Drug Delivery, J. Med. Sci. 2009; 9(6):249-256.
47. Fischer S., Foreg C., Merkle P.H., Gander B., Chitosan Coated Plga-Microspheres-A Modular System for Targeting Drug Delivery, European Cells and Materials. 2004; 7:11-12.
48. Ghulam M., Mahmood A., Naveed A., Fatima R.A., Comparative study of various microencapsulation techniques. Effect of polymer viscosity on microcapsule characterstics, Pak.J.Sci.2009; 22 (3):291-300.

49. Tamizharasi S., Rathi C.J., Rathi., Formulation and Evaluation of Pentoxyfylline-Loaded Poly (ε- caprolactone) Microspheres, Indian Journal of pharmaceutical Sciences. 2008; 70(3):333- 337.
50. Kataria S, Akanksha M, Premjeet S, Bilandi A, Kapoor B. Microsphere: A Review. International Journal of Research in Pharmacy and Chemistry. 2011; 1(4): 1184-1198 105.Kalyan S, Sharma P. Recent Advancement in Chitosan Best Formulation and Its Pharmaceutical Application. Pelagia Research Library. 2010;1(3):195-210.
51. Prasad B, Gupta V, Devana N, Jayasurya K. Microspheres as Drug Delivery Systems: A Review. Journal of Global Trends in Pharmaceutical Science. 2014; 5(3): 1961-1972.
52. Kalyan Shweta, Sharma Parmod Kumar. Recent Advancement in Chitosan Best Formulation and Its Pharmaceutical Application. Pelagia Research Library. 1(3), 2010, 195-210.
53. Gholap SB, Banarjee SK, Gaikwad DD, Jadhav SL and Borat RM. Hollow microsphere: a review, International Journal of Pharmaceutical Sciences Review and Research.
2010; 1:10-15.
54. Sudha Mani T and Naveen Kumar K. At preparation and evaluation of ethyl cellulose microspheres of ibuprofen for sustained drug delivery International Journal of Pharma Research and Development. 2010;2(8):120-121.
55. Nano BC, Sunny MC and Jayakrishnan A. Cross-linked chitosan microspheres: Preparation and evaluation as a matrix for the controlled release of pharmaceuticals. J Pharm Pharmacol. 1992; 44:283-286.
56. Parmar Harshad, Bakliwal, Sunil at al. Different Method of Evaluation of Mucoadhesive Microsphere, International Journal of Applied Biology and Pharmaceutical Technology. 2010;1(3):1164-1165.
57. Kavita Kunchu, Raje Veera Ashwani et al. Albumin Microspheres: A Unique system as drug delivery carriers for non- steroidal anti-inflammatory drugs. 2010;5(2):12.
58. Kalyan Shweta, Sharma Parmod Kumar et al. Recent Advancement in Chitosan Best Formulation and Its Pharmaceutical Application. Pelagia Research Library. 2010;1(3):195-210.
59. Corrigan l. Owen and Healy Marie Anne. Surfactants in Pharmaceutical Products and Systems "Encyclopedia of Pharmaceutical Technology" 3rd edition, 2003 volume 1, edited by James Swarbrick Informa healthcare Inc. P.NO – 35.

60. T. Omkar, M. Alagusundaram, S.C. Madhu, K. Umashankari, V.B. Attuluri, C. Lavanya, B. Ramkanth, Microspheres as a novel drug delivery system, Int J of Chem Tech and Res, 3(1),2009,526-534.
61. N.R. Patel, D.A. Patel, P.D Bharadia, V. Pandya, V. Modi, Microsphere as a novel drug deliver, Int J of Pharm & Life Sci,2(8),2011,992-997.
62. V.V. Prasanth, A.C. Moy, S.T. Mathew, R. Mathapan, Microspheres: an overview, Int J of Pharm & Biomedical Sci, 2(2),2011,332-338.
63. P. Chandrawanshi, H. Patidar, Magnetic microspheres: as a targeted drug delivery, J of Pharm Res, 2(5), 2009, 964-966.
64. Chawla, P. Gupta, V. Karadia, A.K. Bansal, Gastro retention - A means to address
65. regional variability in intestinal drug absorption, Pharm Tech ,27(2),2003,50-68.
66. S.P. Gholap, S.K. Banrjee, D.D Gaikwad, S.L. Jadhav, R.M. □orat, Hollow microspheres: A Review, Int J of Pharm Sci Review and Res ,1(1),2010,74-79.
67. U. Hafeli, R.W. Atcher, C.E. Morris, B. Beresford, J.L. Humm, R.M. Macklis, Polymeric radiopharmaceutical delivery systems, Radioactivity & Radiochemistry, 3, 1992,11-14.
68. Jain, A.K. Panda, D.K. Majumdar, Eudragit S100 Entrapped Insulin Microspheres for Oral Delivery, AAPS Pharm Sci Tech, 6 (1), 2005, 101-107. Orienti I, K Aiedeh E.
69. Bertasi and V. Zecchi. Indomethacin loaded chitosan microspheres, correlation between the erosion as drug Carriers: a review. Journal of Pharmaceutical Sciences and Research. 2009;1(2):1-12.
70. Sinha V R, Bansal K, Kaushik R, Kumria R, Trehan A. Polycaprolactone microspheres and nanospheres, International Journal of Pharmaceutics (2004) 278 1–23.
71. Sinha V R, Singla A K, Wadhawan S, Kaushik R, Kumria R, Bansal K, Dhawan S, Chitosan microspheres as a potential carrier for drugs, International Journal of Pharmaceutics274;2004, 1–33.
72. Jayaprakash S, Halith S M, Mohamed Firthouse P U, Kulaturanpillai K, Abhijith, Nagarajan M. Preparation and evaluation of biodegradable microspheres of methotrexate. Asian J Pharm,3;2009,26-9.
73. Parikh D, Spray drying as a granulation Technique; In: Handbook of Pharmaceutical Granulation Technology, Drugs and the Pharmaceutical Sciences. New York, Marcel Dekker 1997, 75-96.

74. Swarbrick b j, Spray drying and Spray Congealing of Pharmaceuticals, In: Encyclopedia of Pharmaceutical Technology, Marcel Dekker. 1992, 207-221. 14 Koff US patent
(March21963) 3,080,292.
75. John P M, Becker C H, J. pharm sci. (1968)57, 584. 16 He P, Davis S S. Illum, L, Chitosan microspheres prepared by spray drying. Int, J. Pharm,187;1999a,53–65.
76. Giunchedi P, Conti B, Maggi L, Conte U, Cellulose acetate butyrate and polycaprolactone for keto proton spray-dried microsphere preparation J Microencapsul.11;1994, 381– 393.
77. Bogataj M, Mrhar A, Grabnar I, Rajtman Z, Bukovec P, Srcic S, Urleb U, The influence of magnesium stearate on the characteristics of mucoadhesive microspheres, Micro encapsule J pharm. sci. 17;2000,499–508.
78. Lim S T, Martin G P, Berry D J, Brown M B, Preparation and evaluation of the in vitro drug release properties and muco adhesion of novel microspheres of hyaluronic acid and chitosan J Control Rel. 66;2000),281–292.
79. Berthold A, Cremer K, Kreuter J, Influence of crosslinking on the acid stability and physicochemical properties of chitosan microspheres. STP Pharm. Sci,6;1996 b,358–364.
80. Alagusundaram M, Madhu S C C, Umashankari K, Attuluri V B, Lavanya C, Ramkanth S, Microspheres as a Novel Drug Delivery System, Chemtech,13;2009, 526-534.
81. Li Y P, Machida T Y, Sanan T, Nagai T, Preparation of chitosan microspheres containing fluorouracil using the 'dryin-oil' method and its release characteristics. STP Pharm. Sci. 1;1991,363–368.
82. Kyotani S, Nishioka Y, Okamura M, Tanaka T, Miyazaki M, Ohnishi S, Yamamoto Y, Ito K, Ogiso T, Tanada S, A study of embolizing materials for chemo-embolization therapy of hepatocellular carcinoma antitumor effect of cis diamine di chloroplatinum(II) albumin microspheres, containing chitin and treated with chitosan on rabbits with VX2 hepatic tumors. Chem. Pharm. Bull. (Tokyo), 40;1990,2814–2816.
83. Jameela S R, Jayakrishnan A, Glutaraldehyde crosslinked chitosan microspheres as a long acting biodegradable drug delivery vehicle: studies on the in vitro release of mitoxantrone. Biomaterials 16;1995, 769–775.
84. Hassan E E, Parish R C, Gallo J M, Optimized formulation of magnetic chitosan microspheres containing the anticancer agent, oxantrazole. Pharm. Res.9;1992, 390–397.

85. Shah S, Qaqish R, Patel V, Amiji M, Evaluation of the factors influencing stomach-specific delivery of antibacterial agents for Helicobacter pylori infection. J. Pharm. Pharmacol.51;1999, 667–672.
86. Shiraishi S, Imai T, Otagiri M, Controlled release of indomethacin by chitosan–polyelectrolyte complex: optimization and in vivo/in vitro evaluation J. Control Rel,25;1993, 217–225.
87. Murata Y, Miyamoto E, Kawashima S, Additive effect of chondroitin sulfate and chitosan on drug release from calcium induced alginate gel beads. J. Control Rel,38;1996,101–108.
88. Bayomi M A, al-Suwayeh S A, el-Helw A M, Mesnad A F, Preparation of casein–chitosan microspheres containing diltiazem hydrochloride by an aqueous coacervation technique. Pharm. Acta Helv.73;1998,187–192.
89. Jameela S R, Kumary T V, Lal A V, Jayakrishnan A, Progesterone-loaded chitosan microspheres: a long acting bio-degradable controlled delivery system. J. Control Rel.52;1998,17–24.
90. Huang H, Tian H, Li X, Zhao G, Hypoglycemic effect of chitosan-micro capsulated insulin on the blood glucose level of streptozotocin-diabetic Wistar rats. Sheng Wu Yi Xue Gong Cheng Xue Za Zhi,18; 2008, 425–427.
91. Lamprecht A, Ubrich N, Hombreiro Perez M, Lehr C,Hoffman M, Maincent P, Influences of process parameters on nanoparticle preparation performed by a double emulsion pressure homogenization technique. Int. J. Pharm. 196;2000, 177–182.
92. Shah S, Qaqish R, Patel V, Amiji M, Evaluation of the factors influencing stomach-specific delivery of antibacterial agents for Helicobacter pylori infection. J. Pharm. Pharmacol. 51;1999, 667–672.
93. Giunchedi P, Genta I, Conti B, Muzzarelli R A, Conte U, Preparation and characterization of ampicillin loaded methyl pyrrolidinone chitosan and chitosan microspheres. Bio-materials,19; 1998,157–161.
94. Hejazi R, Amiji M, Stomach-specific anti-H. pylori therapy. II. Gastric residence studies of tetracycline-loaded chitosan microspheres in gerbils. Pharm. Dev.Technol,8;2003, 253–262.
95. Farraj N F, Johansen B R, Davdi S S, Illum L, Nasal administration of insulin using bio-adhesive microspheres as a delivery system. J. Control. Release.13;1990,253-261.
96. Illum L, Farraj N F, Davis S S, Johansen B R, O'Hagan D T Investigation of the nasal absorption of biosynthetic human growth hormone in sheep-use of a bio-adhesive

microsphere delivery system. Int. J. Pharm 63; 1990,207- 211.

97. Critchley H,Davis S S, Farraj N F, Illum L, Nasal absorption of desmopressin in rats and sheep-effect of a bioadhesive microsphere delivery system. J. Pharm. Pharmacol.46;1994,651-656.
98. Akiyama Y, Nagahara N, Novel formulation approaches to oral mucoadhesive drug delivery system. In: Mathiowitz E, Chickering DE, Lehr CM. (Eds.), Bio-adhesive Drug Delivery Systems-Fundamentals, Novel Approaches and Development 1998. 477–505.
99. Illum L, Farraj N F, Fisher A N, Gill J, Miglietta M, Benedetti L M, Hyaluronic acid ester microsphere as a nasal delivery system for insulin. J. Control. Release,29;1994, 332- 334.
100. Akiyama Y, Yoshioka M, Horibe H, Inada Y, Hirai S, Kitamori N, Toguchi H, Anti-hypertensive effect of oral controlled release microspheres containing an ACE inhibitor (Delapril hydrochloride) in rats. J. Pharm. Pharmacol 46;1994, 661-665.

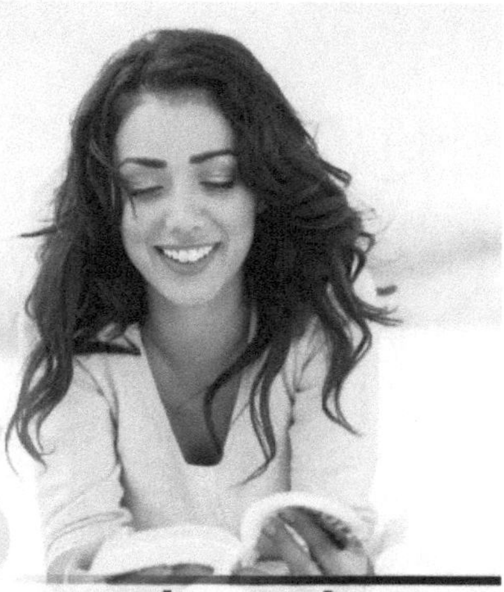

FSC
www.fsc.org
MIX
Papier | Fördert
gute Waldnutzung
FSC® C083411

Kolibri 360 GmbH
Ferdinand-Jühlke-Straße 7
99095 Erfurt, Deutschland
produktsicherheit@kolibri360.de

Druck:
CPI Druckdienstleistungen GmbH
im Auftrag der
Kolibri 360 GmbH
Ferdinand-Jühlke-Str. 7
99095 Erfurt